KATHLEEN GRIFFIN is a writer and an award-winning BBC broadcaster. She lectures on forgiveness and runs forgiveness workshops for those who want to be free of the traumatic events in their past. She is currently working on her fourth book, a memoir of her French family. Griffin lives in London.

The
Forgiveness
Formula

The
Forgiveness
Formula

How to Let Go of Your Pain
and Move On with Life

Kathleen Griffin

MARLOWE & COMPANY
NEW YORK

For Nelson Mandela and the people of South Africa

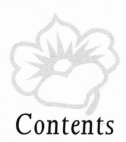

Contents

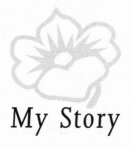

My Story

I HAD JUST TURNED eleven when I was abducted. It was the end of my first month in middle school and I was going to a party at school. There'd been an argument at home about what I should wear—my parents had insisted that I wear my school uniform while I knew everyone would be in casual clothes. But the uniform had cost so much money. I knew how proud they were of my passing the entrance exam and getting a scholarship to the best school in the area, so I gave in. I was allowed to wear some patterned tights that were all the rage.

I waited at the bus stop as usual, opposite the church we went to every Sunday. The bus took ages and I was worried about being late. Then a car pulled up and a man who looked to be in his late twenties or early thirties got out. He asked me where I was going, and having been brought up to be polite to adults, I told him. He said he'd take me there. I hesitated, hoping the bus would come and knowing I was already late. He was pleasant and said he'd make sure he got me there on time.

For a mile or so we chatted about school, etc., and then he asked me how old I was. I didn't want to appear like a baby, so I said thirteen. "What a lovely age," he said, which I thought was a strange response, but adults were always saying strange things. We were just pulling up to a traffic circle when he said, "Hold on to that, would you," quite cheerfully. I looked down and saw that he had taken his penis out of his pants. I didn't know what to do. I wasn't scared exactly, just surprised that he should say it so casually while he continued driving. So I put what seemed a tiny hand round his penis and it was hard—I had never seen an erect penis before—and after about a minute he groaned and got out a handkerchief and wiped himself and then went on chatting happily and said he would make sure I got to the party on time.

Then we came to a fork in the road and he took the turning away from the town and stopped the car after about a hundred yards. By now I was feeling scared and he told me angrily that he had promised to get me to the party and he would. He said that if I ever told anyone what had happened, we would both be in a lot of trouble and that he would go to prison, and that I would go to prison too, for getting in the car with him.

By now, I was really scared because although I couldn't see what I had done wrong, I was sure he was right that I would be in a lot of trouble if anyone ever found out. All I wanted was to get away and get to the party. The bus I should have caught came past on the main road and I said, "I have to get to the party or I'll get yelled at." Then he leaned over and tried to kiss me. I knew then that what he was doing was wrong, that grown-ups didn't kiss children like he was trying to, with his tongue in my mouth, and I started to cry. Suddenly he got angry again and told me not to cry; he'd said that he'd take me to the party and he would—we were just going for a little drive first.

It was then that I knew with absolute certainty and more clearly than I have ever known anything in my life, before or since, that he was going to kill me. My whole body went cold and I imagined for a moment how my family would feel if I were dead, how sad they would be. And at that moment I knew that I had to choose. To go along with him, stay in the car—and that meant I would die—or somehow to try to escape. I thought about it fairly calmly for what seemed like hours but was in fact two or three minutes. Then I chose, quite deliberately, to live.

It seemed like my mind went into overdrive. He tried to start the car but the back wheel was spinning in mud. He reached over and locked my side, told me to stay put and got out to find something to put under the back wheel. Again I knew I had to make a decision, to stay put and die, or to live. I looked in the side mirror and saw him bent over the back wheel. I quietly unlocked the door, eased myself out of the car, and started running for my life. He shouted and tried to grab me as I went past, but I brushed him off, running as fast as I could to the main road where there were cars.

He came after me but stopped when we got to the main road and I ran up the hill to the bus stop and a bus came almost immediately. I got on and sat down and by the time we passed the junction he was gone. My heart was beating so fast I thought everyone on the bus must be able to hear it. It felt like it was going to burst out of my body.

After about ten minutes I began to calm down but now felt terrified he was going to come after me; I kept looking out of the window to see if he was following the bus. I was now very late for the party, which would be in full swing. What should I do? Should I tell someone what had happened? I started crying but no one on the bus took any notice.

I got off at the school stop and ran into school, looking over my shoulder all the time in case the man had followed me. Then in the corridor I met a teacher who told me to hurry along as the party had already started. Then she stopped me and looked more closely at me and asked what was wrong. It was clear I had been crying.

I was about to blurt out what had happened when I had another moment of being aware that I had two choices. It felt like a road forking ahead in two different directions into the future. Just like being in the car, when I had to choose to live or die, now I had to choose to tell or keep silent. This was my first month in a new school. The man had said I would be in terrible trouble if I told anyone what happened, that I might go to prison. But this was my one chance: if I didn't tell this teacher right now, no one would believe me later.

Yet if I did tell her, I knew there would be a terrible commotion. That for my whole time at school I would be labeled as the girl this had happened to, and what I wanted most of all was to melt into the crowd and not draw attention to myself. I wasn't sure anyone would believe me, but I knew that somehow I would be blamed. Somehow it would be my fault, for getting into the car in the first place, for touching his penis . . .

The teacher was kind enough but getting impatient for an answer, and pressed me again to tell her what was wrong, asking me why I had worn my uniform on a Saturday. That was when I decided. I was already different from the other girls whose parents had known not to send them to school in uniform. Did I want to cause a huge fuss and be pointed out by everyone? I knew then that I didn't. I muttered about being upset at missing the bus and being late and being forced to wear my uniform by my parents, by which time she had had enough and kindly ushered me into the school hall where the games were in full swing.

The rest of the afternoon passed in a dream. I played the games, ate the hot dogs and Jell-O, and drank the lemonade, but it was as if I was watching a film. I saw the other girls and teachers and myself through a glass partition; the real me was somewhere else. And when I went to the bathroom, I washed my hands again and again, sure that I could still smell the man on me.

When I got home I realized that this was my last chance to say anything, that if I didn't tell my parents now, I would have to keep what had happened a secret forever. My mom and dad met me at the door, eager to know how the party had been, if I had enjoyed myself and made any new friends. I felt how much they wanted everything at the new school to go well, how important it was to them that I should make the best of things. And I said nothing.

It wasn't until many years later that I felt able to tell someone—the man I was in love with. I wasn't sure how he would react. Luckily he was great, and once I had told him the story it felt like it had been put to rest. But years after that, I started having flash-backs of what had happened and I realized that I hadn't dealt with it at all, but simply reburied the memory. And that I was so angry that I still wanted to kill my attacker. Most of all, however, with the fear and the anger, came the knowledge that I did not want to feel like that for the rest of my life. So began my journey of forgiveness.

The
Forgiveness
Formula

PART 1

The Forgiveness Path

1

Choosing Forgiveness

If we could read the secret history of our enemies, we would find
in each person's life, sorrow and suffering enough to disarm all
hostility.

HENRY LONGFELLOW

*F*ORGIVENESS IS A journey, and in picking up this book you have
taken the first step. It may be that you have been thinking of
letting go of a hurt that needs forgiveness for many years. You may
simply be fed up with carrying the burden of not forgiving. Or it
may never have occurred to you before, but you somehow felt
drawn to this book.

Whatever the reason, you are already engaged with the process
of forgiveness, and this book will give you a practical step-by-step
guide through the difficulties. We will also discuss some of the
more complicated issues raised by forgiveness and how we can
begin to deal with them.

We all have people we need to forgive. It may not be for sins as
grave as that recounted in my story, but all of us have at least one person who we feel has done us real wrong. It may be a parent, sibling,

lover, or friend. They may be long dead or very much alive. Until we learn to forgive them, we carry in our heart the pain that person has caused us. And the more wrong they did us, the more pain we carry.

Forgiveness has been a hard lesson in my own life. It took me decades to realize what a corrosive effect withholding forgiveness had had on me. When I did, I had no choice but to start, however reluctantly, on the path of forgiveness. That first step—choosing forgiveness—is a big one, so let's look at what it might mean.

Close your eyes. Just imagine for a moment what it would be like to forgive. Just for once put all the good reasons for not forgiving to one side: however wrong it felt, however much pain it caused, however thoughtless the act, let these reasons drop away from you. Imagine a box as big as you like—put them all in there; don't leave a single reason behind. Now feel, really feel what it is like to have the weight of those reasons for not forgiving hanging round your neck, weighing you down. This book will help you to fill the box and let it go. But the choice is yours at every stage of the journey.

Just picking up this book means that a voice somewhere deep within you is ready to think about it, to give it a try. When you get to the end of Part 1 you may decide there are things that will always be impossible for you to let go of. That's fine. It's not an easy journey and there is no rush. Forgiveness is a process and you will discover that step by step.

- ❧ You cannot forgive until you are ready.
- ❧ You cannot forgive until you are willing.
- ❧ Your forgiveness journey is yours alone—it takes the time it takes.

What would it take to begin the journey?

When we withhold forgiveness, we are often trying to make things the same as they were before we were really badly hurt. Forgiveness is then not an option, because it would seem to deny the injustice of what has been done to us. Ask yourself these questions:

- If you could make people really understand how much you have been hurt, could you imagine letting go?
- If you could punish the person who hurt you, could you let go?
- Was everything fine "before"?

For those of us who have been deeply hurt there is often a "before" and "after." We remember the before as a time without problems. If only we could go back there. Withholding forgiveness is then our way of retaining some power in the situation. It is our way of trying to change the narrative to go back to how things used to be.

To begin the journey of forgiveness we need to give up the hope of things being as they were "before." Things are different. You are different.

Accepting that what happened to you really did happen is the first step. But it is the hardest step of all.

Sometimes we hold on so hard to the hatred, to the unwillingness to let go and forgive, that we become one with the withholding—it becomes who we are.

How could it be different?

- How quickly do you tell "your story" when you meet someone new?
- How often do you think about the person who has done you most wrong? All the time, once a week, once a year?
- How has withholding forgiveness affected other relationships in your life?

Withholding forgiveness certainly fills you with the energy of anger and injustice. In my own case, I buried the memory of being abducted as a child for many years. It was so deeply buried that when I eventually told someone in my early twenties, I was astonished at the depth of anger that I still felt about it. If I could have killed that man I would have done it, happily, without a second thought. That shocked me, too. But I simply couldn't let go of the feeling of passionate anger.

Telling someone and being believed and supported helped a lot, but it was not till another fifteen years had passed and the memories returned as flashbacks that I realized I was still furious and ready to kill him. In the meantime that anger had been put to good use: I had often been involved in defending the underdog and been active in social change. I couldn't bear any form of injustice. It was only much later that I realized that championing the cause of the underdog was my way of trying to make my own voice heard. That I wished that someone had been ready to champion me when I needed it.

Luke was repeatedly sexually abused by a teacher at school and twenty years later went to the police, who arrested the teacher and brought a case against him. For Luke, the idea of clinging to what happened to him makes some sense.

"I think many people hold on because what happens is that often when people commit an offence against us, it touches us deeply. As a society, we don't know how to express or deal with those feelings. The feeling of joy, I've realized, has the same extreme effect as pain does. And what happens is that we all long to be alive, we all long to deeply feel because we were created to feel and so, for some people, the offence committed against them gives them a sense of feeling deeply, of being alive."

Luke has encountered the same emotions of anger and passion in many people who have been sexually abused.

"It gives them a passion, whether it's a passion to be angry about something, or feel joy about something. It's a passion, a sense of 'I am still alive.' In my journey as a survivor of abuse, I have been to different groups, where people sit there and they feel victims and they want to stay victims, because the offence committed has now become their identity. For many people, particularly if the offence has been committed while they were children, it's all they have ever known and to actually lose that, the fear is that 'I will have no identity at all and at least this has given me something to be passionate about.' But there's a time at which that has to be left behind and the other emotions and experiences in life have to be allowed the possibility to bear fruit."

Ethel is ninety-three and hadn't spoken to her brother, who lives half a mile away, for more than forty years. "I can't even remember what we fell out about but we shan't speak this side of the grave," she said and sent a chill down my spine. She could barely remember why they didn't speak (something to do with a disagreement about a family funeral) but they had both hung on all these years to the bitterness. They would occasionally bump into each other in the street and pretend they didn't know one another.

But the wound wasn't healed: she cried when she told me the story. There was a terrible mixture of feelings; she was proud and determined but also confused that she couldn't really remember what it was about. One thing was clear to her though: it was impossible to put right—who was going to make the first move?

Ethel died a year after we had this conversation and she still hadn't spoken to her brother. He came to her funeral and was in tears as the coffin was taken out. Now there was no chance of reconciliation —they had both been too stubborn to make the first move.

Sometimes the hurt is all that is left of a relationship and it has been clung to so tenaciously that it has come to symbolize the relationship itself. At least you have the pain to connect you. To let go of that then becomes impossible because it seems as though there would be no relationship left. So Ethel went to her grave not speaking to a brother over a half-remembered grievance.

Sometimes it is the death itself that is hard to forgive. When Betty's mother died of cancer, Betty was surprised to find how hard it was to forgive her for dying. As an only child, whose father had died when she was a teenager, Betty felt that her mother had left her on her own.

"I felt very unforgiving toward her, because I felt she'd gone away from me very suddenly—she died four months after she was diagnosed. Though in some ways that gave me time to prepare with her for her death, of course there are many things that you can never prepare for, so in that sense I remained unforgiving."

Betty was surprised by this anger. "When my father died I was that much younger and I can't recall feeling so angry. It doesn't sound logical, but of course you can be angry at the injustice of it all and to me it was a very unjust situation that somebody I loved very dearly, for that to be taken away from her and from me. So in an odd way I did feel very angry at her, being left; she was my mother and she had left me on my own. The Christmas after she died I had a bout of flu and I felt really angry toward her because she wasn't around to help me. Sounds very selfish, but *that's how I felt. I was regressing into childhood, remembering my mother being so loving and of course that was gone, so I felt very angry."*

Betty went through the grieving process and although it was a very painful few years, she has now come out the other side and been able to let go of the anger she felt at being left.

"When I've forgiven the things that I think went wrong in the relationship with my mother I have felt much, much better. Like a great weight, letting go. While you are at a point where it is difficult, it usually means you keep going back to the period or the incident that made you resentful. If I can decide that's over then I can let it go."

Betty had a good relationship with her mother. Anger at the loved one who has died is a recognized part of the grieving process, but it can feel inappropriate and embarrassing to the loved ones left behind. Yet by holding on to the anger at the person who has died, we may feel that they are not completely gone, that some part of them is still here with us.

Of course if the relationship with the dead person was not good while they were alive, much is generally unresolved at the point of death. It is only in films and novels that deathbed scenes of forgiveness take place. In real life it is much more likely that the grudges and grievances will be taken to the grave, which leaves the people left behind with a strong sense of things not being resolved. Hanging on to the anger loops us back into "not letting them get away with it." We feel that we are alive and having the final say in the argument. Even if there is no one left to argue with.

From victim to victor

Sometimes it feels impossible to find a way back to forgiveness. It's as though you are in a maze and have lost the thread of the way out. Taking the first steps on the forgiveness journey can seem impossible. But would you want to go to your grave as Ethel did, holding firm to a resentment of which she couldn't even remember the origins?

Withholding forgiveness can be about transferred pain—the need to find someone to blame. This is particularly true when something terrible has happened. So should we ever stand firm and not forgive? Is it ever a valid choice?

"Forgiveness is costly, it is painful, it's difficult, and it is a choice. Why is it sometimes people cannot forgive? One of the reasons, sometimes, is because nobody has acknowledged, reverenced, recognized the story of what has happened, sufficiently deeply."

Father Michael Lapsley knows what he is talking about. He is an Anglican priest who was involved in the anti-apartheid struggle in South Africa. In 1990 he was sent a letter bomb by the South African authorities. He lost both his hands and an eye in the explosion. Father Lapsley spoke at the Forgiveness conference at the Findhorn Foundation in Scotland in 1999 and emphasized the need for making the transition from victim to survivor and eventually to victor. He spoke about the fact that remaining filled with anger and hatred would keep him entrenched in the role of victim.

Moving from victim to victor means

- not remaining stuck in the narrative of what was done to you;
- choosing to tell the story differently; and
- learning that it doesn't have to stop there.

Father Lapsley makes the crucial distinction between healing and forgiving. He now works with "Healing the Memories" workshops throughout South Africa and he believes it vitally important to Heal and Remember, not Bury and Forget. But he is very clear where he personally stands on forgiveness.

"*Often when I have spoken in different places around the world, I have told my story, as I tell it now, and said I am not filled with hatred and bitterness and pity, and I don't want revenge. Then at the end some nice person is asked to stand up and thank me and they say, 'It's absolutely wonderful! This person is an icon of forgiveness,' and I say, 'I beg your pardon, I haven't mentioned the word forgiveness. I haven't said I have forgiven anybody.' In a sense forgiveness for me isn't on the table, you see, because no one has said to me, 'I did it.'"*

We can only be silent in the face of such suffering. Father Lapsley challenges us to take forgiveness as seriously as he does and shows that it is a long journey, not an easy path. You can only get there when you are ready, when you feel it is time for restitution and reparation for what has happened. If that is not forthcoming, it makes the journey a much longer one. Forgiveness is not easy and it is not straightforward, and anyone who thinks it is has not understood the darker side of what human beings can do to one another.

The one who pursues revenge should first dig two graves.
CHINESE PROVERB

Sometimes we need to withhold forgiveness until we are really ready to let go. And that means letting time heal the wounds or waiting until we come to a fork in the road—one path leading to forgiveness, the other to bitterness.

Clare went through a traumatic break-up of a ten-year marriage. The first she knew that anything was wrong was when she found a note on her kitchen table from her husband telling her that he was leaving.

"For years I held on to the role of victim. I was this person who had acted well in the relationship and had this terrible thing done to them. When I would tell the story, I would see shock on people's faces, reinforcing that it was a terrible thing to do. Several things happened to make me change. A good male friend was driving me to the station one day and asked me if I could imagine a day when I would not need to tell the story. And the terrible thing was, I couldn't. That brought me up short.

And then one day when I was telling the story yet again at another dinner party, I thought, I've become this person—this woman who was left. I don't want it to be my identity. I realized I had come to a fork in the road: I could legitimately assume the identity of 'the woman who was left out of the blue.' Or I could let it go, forgive him, and move on.

It took me years to let go of it completely, but the other day I found myself in a situation where I could have told the story and didn't—and realized that it was well and truly over, that I had no desire to be identified in that way. I am no longer that person."

Clare shows that we can only forgive when the time is right. She needed to hang on to blame, to identify herself as the victim that she in fact was, and to get reinforcement for that role from the outside world. And eventually she came to a fork in the road that we all come to when we travel along the forgiveness highway—I can choose to let go and forgive or go down the lack of forgiveness route. Neither is an easy choice—forgiving involves a letting go that can feel like a tearing of the soul in two.

- ☙ Are you ready to stop telling your story in the old way?
- ☙ Are you ready to be open to the possibility of a new way of telling the same story?
- ☙ What is your fork in the road?

Forgiveness must be an individual decision, freely made

What we can say is that there are some people who have gone through unimaginably dreadful experiences and somehow come to a place of forgiveness. At the same Forgiveness conference in Findhorn, a woman from Rwanda whose whole family, apart from her son, had been massacred, stood up and said, *"Do not pity me. I have forgiven them. Feel sorry for the people who did this."*

She is now working for peace in Rwanda, a region of Africa where whole communities were butchered simply for belonging to the "wrong" ethnic group. Several members of religious orders, both priests and nuns, have been convicted of taking part in the butchery. How can a country begin to heal those wounds with forgiveness? What do you do with the thousands of possible murderers still held in prison? What about the orphan generations; how do you ensure that they do not continue the massacres of revenge when they are old enough? It is enough to make anyone despair, yet this woman is working actively for peace in her own region, having experienced the loss of almost her entire family.

> This is certain, that a man that studieth revenge keeps his
> wounds green, which otherwise would heal and do well.
> FRANCIS BACON

Learning which fights to fight

Sometimes the internal conflicts we have about forgiveness become transferred into fighting in the outside world. It seems so hard to forgive, so easy to take on other causes that need fighting.

Simon is the sort of person who is completely dependable. He is the best friend anyone could want, a rock, the sort of person you could call at four in the morning with a crisis and he would be ready to help without question. The sort of man who recently saw a bunch of teenagers picking a fight and waded in to stop them without hesitation. He sits on several national charitable boards and hates injustice enough to fire off letters and e-mails to the papers and politicians. But he is not someone to have as an enemy. *"It's a gut feeling. I don't feel hurt when someone does something serious to offend me, I bristle. Then I feel if you come into my territory, I will mow you down."*

He always has several ongoing fights on his hands. They seem to fire him with enthusiasm, whether it is taking on a bureaucracy about unfair parking regulations or defending a friend who has lost his benefits or writing to the papers about some international incident. Simon recognizes this trait as a kind of reaction to his father. *"My father would feel hurt forever rather than bear a grudge. I'm different. I don't feel a victim: in a way I'm temperamentally well suited to the vendetta."*

The choice is yours

Withholding forgiveness is painful in a different way—it leads to a hardening of the heart.

No one else can tell you to forgive, or when to forgive. It is completely your choice. Withholding forgiveness is valid for as long as it serves you—for some people it is the essence of what helps them to survive. Those who have not experienced much pain in their lives are often the first to advocate forgiveness, as though it were a moral failing not to forgive. Those people urging easy forgiveness often have no great understanding of the suffering involved in the journey.

This is a judgment call—forgive when you are ready and you can really let go. It might seem that ideally we would do fast-track forgiveness—you hurt me, I forgive you, and that's the end of it. But life is not like that and nor would it be appropriate.

Withholding forgiveness might seem justified in the context of the great evils of the twentieth century. Must the Jews who went through the Holocaust forgive the Nazis? In the face of such evil, it is not for us to make easy and snap judgments. But even in these terrible situations there are certain things we can say about forgiveness.

Most people would agree that it would be impossible to forgive the Nazi who murdered your family in the Holocaust—though some have shown that it is possible. And by extension it may not be possible to forgive anyone who was an enthusiastic supporter of the Nazis. But how far does the blame go? Should you hate all Germans alive at the time? Or simply all Germans, even those born since the war? Or all Germans who will ever be born? Where does the blame stop? And if you are in this situation, do you want your children and grandchildren to feel the same way? Where does the blame end?

One survivor of the Holocaust who had found it possible to forgive, said to another who had not, "*Then you are still there in prison with them.*"

What do you have to gain from not forgiving?

- What do you get out of withholding forgiveness?
- What do you imagine life would be like if you let go?
- How possible does it seem?

- What is the alternative if you don't forgive—what do you imagine your life will be like in ten years' time?
- If you had children, would you want to pass this feeling on to them?

If we withhold forgiveness, it may hurt us in the long run. But let's be clear: forgiveness isn't the easy path; for many of us it's a path we would not have chosen. But we get there when the alternative becomes unbearable. For me, the penny finally dropped when I was walking along a beach one day, on vacation."

I saw a young girl who was about eleven playing on her own quite happily. I found myself looking round to see where her family was and whether there were any threatening characters lurking. And suddenly I was plunged back into flashbacks of my own abduction. That was when I realized that I didn't want to be like this anymore, when the sight of a young girl playing happily on the beach could take me to such a painful place. I had no thought of forgiveness then; it was the last thing on my mind. But I knew that where I was, full of hatred for this man, no longer worked for me. If you had told me then that this first step on the journey would eventually lead me to forgive the man who had abducted me, I wouldn't have believed you.

No one can make that journey for you, no one can take you there, no one can force you to take the first steps on the path. It is such a hard path that you have to be willing to go there yourself, to take the first steps on your own and trust in the process.

If your issues of forgiveness are ones that have been passed down to you through the family narrative, you need to ask yourself some serious questions. Withholding forgiveness is likely to be passed down the generations like a baton in a relay race. It takes courage to say, "This stops here. Now. With me."

One thing is certain: holding on means passing on

Choosing not to forgive may be a valid choice—for the moment. Some of us have such terrible experiences in our lives that it just feels impossible to move on to forgiveness. If something awful has happened to someone we love, it may feel disloyal to forgive the perpetrator, particularly if the person has never been brought to justice. Or it may feel that our identity is tightly wrapped up in what happened to us and that to let go would leave us with just a big hole in our hearts. The act of holding on to the grievance may feel as if that is what helps us get up and survive one more day.

Believe no one who uses the words *must* or *should* when it comes to forgiveness. Father Michael Lapsley is critical of many of the orthodox religions for their attitude to forgiveness, which can heap an additional burden on the victim. If they can't find forgiveness, they are made to feel ashamed for not being spiritual enough.

"But also what does it mean to forgive? Much of the discourse of the faith communities gives the impression that it's glib, cheap, and easy, and many of the preachers who speak about forgiveness I would suggest use it as a weapon against people. They increase their burdens."

It would be impertinent to tell those who have gone through terrible experiences that they must, or should forgive. That they are somehow lacking in moral fiber if they don't, or not as good as those people who do come to forgiveness. It is not for us to judge the path of forgiveness in someone else. We are all on the journey of forgiveness, but some of us have things to forgive which are so painful that it may take years even to be able to begin to look at them with any possibility of change. There are some life events from which it is difficult, if not impossible, to recover, and it is important that we honor that experience. That we acknowledge the huge courage of people who live with the memory of these experiences day to day and still manage to hold on to life.

It took Luke a long time to forgive the man who sexually abused him all those years ago. And it has certainly changed him. He now has a job where he is able to influence policy on child abuse in a large organization. He is making a real difference about the quality of children's lives every day. In the past his anger was turned against himself in various destructive ways. Forgiveness has allowed him to use that sense of anger and injustice as a fuel to change the world.

"What I have noticed myself is that by holding on there is a sense of anger, there is a sense of the injustice that has been done to somebody and you are able to feel that injustice. All I can say is that the anger or the sense of injustice have not been diminished from me at all. Actually, on the contrary, I personally think I have got more in touch with it at a deeper level. But I am free to continue my life and not to remain a victim. Forgiving what has been done to me is saying 'I refuse to remain a slave to what's happened to me. I'm going to go on and become the adult person I was created to be.'"

Let's first look at just what the Forgiveness Formula means:

The Forgiveness Formula

- ⚘ It means completely letting go of the hurt this person has done you.
- ⚘ It means letting go of the hold this narrative has had on your life.
- ⚘ It means getting rid of a piece of baggage that you will no longer have to carry around with you.
- ⚘ It does not mean forgetting what has been done to you.
- ⚘ It does not mean that you do not learn lessons from what happened to you.

The Ten Golden Rules of Forgiveness

1. Forgive and the whole landscape will change.
2. You are the only one who can change—those who have done you wrong have nothing to do with your forgiveness process.
3. You can only forgive when you are ready—it won't work until you are.
4. When you forgive and let go, you change and then the whole world is different.
5. There will always be someone else to forgive, so the better you get at it, the easier life will be.
6. When you forgive the big stuff, you will always have a scar on your heart: that way you won't forget.
7. Sitting on top of the mountain of being in the right is a very lonely place.
8. Think of people you know who can forgive. Now think of those who bear a grudge—which camp would you rather be in?
9. If you can learn to forgive yourself, you are more than halfway there.
10. It is never too late to forgive.

2

Redrawing Your
Forgiveness Map

What could you want that forgiveness cannot give? Do you
want peace? Forgiveness offers it. Do you want happiness, a
quiet mind, a certainty of purpose, and a sense of worth and
beauty that transcends the world? Do you want care and
safety, and the warmth of sure protection always? Do you
want a quietness that cannot be disturbed, a gentleness that
never can be hurt, a deep, abiding comfort, and a rest so perfect it can never be upset? All this forgiveness offers you.

A COURSE IN MIRACLES

E ALL HAVE OUR own personal map of the world. That is the
way that we think the world works, how we situate ourselves in the world. If we need to, we can refer to the map to reassure ourselves that we are where we think we are in the world.

M. Scott Peck in his book *The Road Less Traveled* suggests that when
we want to change our view of the world, it is this map that is up
for grabs, that needs to change. When we feel depressed and unable
to cope with the world, our maps no longer seem to point in the
right direction. It's as though all the reassuring landmarks have been

moved so that nothing makes sense any more. We may travel in one direction, sure that it will take us to where we want to go, only to find that the road is blocked by anger, self-sabotage, or hopelessness. And although we may consult the map, which up until now has always given us the right directions in life, it no longer works. We are lost.

Forgiveness involves redrawing our map of the world. But it's not just a question of working out some new grid references. When we change our view of the world as radically as forgiveness demands, we are traveling to another country where eventually the new map will make much more sense and the road will be smoother.

If you think of it as going to a new country, without speaking the language, with no money or credit cards and no means of transport, you will get some idea of how scary the journey may be. But pretty soon you will learn the words for *please* and *thank you* and *hello* and *goodbye* and find that the locals are not as frightening as you first thought. You will learn enough to get by on by working hard at your map, and then you will find yourself at the top of a hill with a fantastic view of the countryside you still have to travel through.

Your family tree of forgiveness

We are now going to make a map of your current state of forgiveness. Get yourself a big piece of paper. This is the family tree of forgiveness that you have been navigating with so far, your ancestral map. It has been handed down to you through the generations, as carefully as any other family heirloom. This is your family's way of doing things—its language of forgiveness, which you were taught from the moment you appeared in the family.

Draw a circle in the middle to represent yourself and various bubbles coming off it to show other influences in your life: parents, grandparents, siblings. Are there family stories that were handed down the generations about family conflicts, grudges, feuds, long bitter rows, resolutions, forgiveness?

What image of forgiveness did you grow up with and where did it come from? What other influences about forgiveness were there in your life—perhaps church or school? Jot down the stories alongside the bubbles and you will gradually see a pattern emerging. Jot down anything that may be relevant about forgiveness: for example, Grandpa bore grudges, or had several people he never spoke to after falling out with them. Build up your own family map of forgiveness gradually, over several days. Once you begin looking at the map and thinking about it, you will be surprised at the family traditions that come up.

Forgiveness is like any other tradition in a family—parts of the family will have stories to tell about forgiveness that may have been passed down the generations, all with one common aim—to let you know "this is the way we do things." As a child you learn your family stories by osmosis. If you hear the stories often enough, they become your narrative too, until you are ready to pass them along to the next generation.

It is very rare for families to question their stories. They are generally accepted as the true family history. Families are also good at assimilating new stories. When a family member marries, the new partner will bring their own family narrative of forgiveness to the table and the family will have to work out a mixture of these two stories. Often one side will be stronger than the other and may dominate the story. You are the product of these stories of forgiveness

stretching back generations, which form your own individual forgiveness family tree.

In general it is the dramas and catastrophes that become enshrined
as family stories, the ones that get added on to and exaggerated with
each retelling, until they become mythic.

But in most families there is also someone who understands the
importance of forgiveness. They probably didn't have anywhere
near as high status as the grudge bearers and revenge seekers. But
they are also important for your map. So now ask yourself if there
is or was anyone in your family who was good at forgiveness?
What influence did they have? Mark them on your map.

Changing the script

It seems to me that some of us are called to be different from what
has gone on in our past family narratives of forgiveness. It is as
though God (or the universe, if you prefer) creates a person in the
family for whom the familiar pattern of withholding forgiveness
no longer works.

Tina has always been aware of a desire to change the family narrative of forgiveness. Her family had a pattern of holding on to
grudges and passing them down to the next generation. But she was
different. *"I wanted to change it. From as early as I could remember, I wanted to
change things. And make them better."*

For her the process was painful and she tried several different
approaches. *"Initially I tried to do it by talking to them and that caused more
hassle! Or by writing to them and in writing to them at times when I hadn't clearly
integrated the issues properly myself and so I was writing with a blaming tone or a
judgmental tone or a God-like tone, like 'I know what is right and you don't,' which*

would just provoke further anger, of course. But eventually I had to make a lot of physical space between me and them and I had to start not expecting anything and trying to learn that they owed me nothing, absolutely nothing.

I had no right to expect them to behave in any particular way, so therefore by making as much physical space I was also preparing psychological space. I also tried to be as constructively forthcoming and open as possible. I reached out to them; some of them had children so I would reach out to them through their children. I began to understand why they thought the way they were thinking."

Tina did the opposite of her family narrative: she worked hard at building bridges of communication. "I had to eat humble pie on lots of levels and tried to be friends again. I have a better space around it now; I expect very little from any of them actually now so it makes it easier."

Betty was very conscious that she was in danger of taking on her mother's narrative of forgiveness, which was being a victim and martyr and holding on to grievances for many years. "I'd be very good at holding on; one of my boyfriends used to call it my little black book. I'd store up grudges and he'd say, 'Oh that's another mark in your little black book, is it?' I'd say, 'Yes,' and I meant it very seriously. It could be very trivial like people not picking clothes up off the floor, or more serious—someone arriving late or letting me down. I'd just mentally make a note of the wrong that they had done me and derive great pleasure from it. Until, and this would happen with friends or partners, until I'd decide, 'OK, that's it. I can't stand to be with you.' So I'd store all those things up. Over a period of time enough black marks would accumulate that I would think—OK, that's it. It wouldn't get worked out, because to work it out would deprive me of the moral high ground so they would just cut off."

Betty has changed, though. Partly by going through the grieving process over her mother's death, she realized that it is important for her not to withhold forgiveness. "I don't do that any more because I realized that a good relationship means that you discuss these issues. If a relationship is worth staying in, whether it is a friend or partner, you discuss them and you hear *what the other person has got to say. And you may well not be in the right, you may be in the wrong yourself and I'm learning that you're not always a saint, you're not always the person sinned against. It's a useful lesson to learn, which is what I think I have been doing."*

All I know is this isn't working any more

So what makes you want things to be different? Just what makes you stand out from all those generations that went before and didn't change? They accepted the family map of forgiveness they had been handed and passed it down to the next generation. What brings you to the point of wanting it to change?

More often than not it's a crisis. A death or a relationship break-up highlights feelings that are normally hidden. Your traditional way of dealing with things doesn't work and you are left flailing around. But this must have happened in the past too. Your ancestors will have had terrible events happen in their lives. But the family narrative of forgiveness was so strong that they couldn't pull away from it, however hard they tried. But maybe they married someone who was slightly different, or managed to move away so the pull of the family was not quite as strong in the next generation, or maybe they brought you up to have the energy to be different.

Whatever the reason, you right here and right now have been given the wonderful chance to do it differently, to change the story.

We all have different ways of not dealing with the crises that come up in our lives—unsuitable affairs, getting really drunk, taking drugs, zoning out in front of the television, eating extra-large tubs of ice cream.

We also know all too well that they just numb the pain, which may be all we want, to start with. But eventually there's a voice somewhere saying, "This isn't working. We need to change." The thought of change can be so scary that we can ignore the voice for years, burying it under layers and layers of inappropriate drinking/sex/tubs of ice cream.

Life shrinks or expands in proportion to one's courage.

ANAÏS NIN

Is there a voice trying to be heard?

- Can you hold a grudge longer than you can hold your breath underwater?
- Do your problems get bottled up and buried beneath several layers of concrete?
- Does the same issue come up again and again in your relationship/family/wider world?
- Do you feel that nobody listens, no matter how loud you shout?
- Is cold silence/sulking your way of dealing with arguments?

Forgiveness is about opening your heart. We decide to change when something in our lives clicks, and the way we used to operate no longer works. Tony had to deal with the death of his brother. His family story gave him nowhere to go. *"In my family forgiving took place quite easily, but I think our problem was that it was done so easily, that things were not worked out or discussed and became repetitive."*

Chloe realized she was affected by her family pattern: *"Grudge is definitely the capital letter in my map, a very deeply seated bitterness, but never* addressed and always with the attitude that it was justified. The feeling that it's got nothing to do with me; the other person can't be forgiven. Even if they do try, even if they try really, really hard to make amends, that grudge will come back. It's never dealt with, you never let go of it. Relationships are not easy in my family and eventually it resurfaces, it always comes back."

And the effect of the family forgiveness map on her life? "I bear grudges, lots and lots of grudges and they go on for years. They've really bothered me because I practice Buddhism and one of the principles is cause and effect, and you realize that at some stage you need to look at yourself and analyze what kind of causes you are making in order to see what is happening in your life. And grudges are probably not very positive so I just wanted to understand them a little better!"

Chloe could trace her family pattern directly back to her grandmother. "My grandmother would say that she didn't mind something, that it was all forgiven, when actually it was eating her up and it was always tiny little things that would just come back over and over again."

Linda drew her family tree of forgiveness and found, "On my father's side the forgiveness narrative was isolation, the ability to cast out, and blame, and bearing a grudge was important. On my mother's side the story was an inability to forgive herself and a profound lack of self-worth."

So Linda had a combination of the isolation and blame from her father and a lack of self-worth, hanging onto her identity as a victim and being unable to forgive herself. Put those together and Linda had inherited a combination that made forgiveness pretty difficult. Her two brothers no longer spoke to her, had cast her out of the family. One of them had died the year before and even on his deathbed had refused to see her to try and come to some sort of reconciliation.

Sue was having serious problems in her marriage. Her husband had had an affair several years ago and though they were still together, she was finding it impossible to forgive him. She was now thinking about staying until her children left home and then leaving the marriage. The whole topic was upsetting to her and she burst into tears as soon as she began talking about it.

Sue drew her map and was puzzled. Her father had had a quick temper but was otherwise quiet. She drew question marks around her mother and seemed to have difficulty describing how her mother reacted. She finally said, "*She just puts up with stuff.*" She did remember being told about her grandfather bearing deep grudges.

At religious school she had been given a strong sense of sin and guilt and punishment. But what was strongest in her map was silence and absence, and after a while she realized that she hadn't ever been given a map of forgiveness. No wonder that when she needed a map herself, to deal with her husband's infidelity, she felt completely lost.

Laura was in the middle of an acrimonious split with her husband of ten years; they had very young children. "*I felt very aggrieved and it was running my life; that was all I felt, that was all I thought about. I felt very depressed and very unhappy, and incredibly full of anger toward this person for what I perceived he had done to me. I felt he had demolished my self-confidence over a great number of years and ground me to a pulp, emotionally. It had reached a point where I felt I was being destroyed as a person. I realized that I couldn't ever really be happy again in the present or the future if I didn't forgive him. I realized also that my self-esteem and forgiveness were linked.*"

Having two very young children meant that she would need to continue to see her partner and be involved with him around all the issues of childcare, and Laura didn't want the animosity to affect her children.

When she drew her forgiveness family tree, Laura found her family didn't talk very much about difficult issues, that they bottled things up. So the map she had inherited wasn't helpful when she was confronted with a situation where she could no longer bottle things up in her marriage but had to uncork all of them.

Some families find it very hard to deal with emotionally difficult situations and the unspoken and unresolved builds up in the family unit like a pressure cooker until something has to give. This was very much the case in Luke's family.

"I was taught very little about forgiveness in my family. It was the usual domestic setting particularly where arguments were concerned. Tempers were flaring; normally my father would instigate a fight, my mother would try and remain calm and when she eventually flew off the handle my father would walk out and lock himself in the bathroom leaving myself and my siblings feeling as though we were walking on eggshells."

It's the emotional giant pink elephant in the middle of the room that everyone can see but no one mentions. Because if you don't mention it, the giant pink elephant doesn't exist. Or if it does, it will just get up and go of its own accord. But of course it's not a great model of forgiveness as a narrative for the children.

"What would happen is that eventually my father would leave the bathroom and he would walk around miserable for a couple of days and then somehow things would almost become balanced again. So the whole topic of forgiveness was not something that was discussed, spoken of, and certainly not publicly practiced within my own family setting."

Trying to redraw the map

Often the partners we choose are a watered-down version of what we have experienced at home. Or a better version. Or a version that is trying to change. So Linda married someone who *"didn't engage and was isolated and had his guard up, but was good at defending me from* my own family." Sue married someone she describes as a *"nice guy but who can't talk in any deep way about his emotions."'* Another version of silence and absence.

Sometimes we suddenly wake up to a pattern, seeing it clearly in other family members. One day, a cousin Linda was close to called her to tell her that his mother had died. Jack was upset because his sister, who had always neglected their mother, was now taking over the funeral arrangements in a way his mother would have hated. Jack felt he could do nothing right—and was being isolated and blamed in a familiar way. Linda could see the family pattern reproducing itself in her cousin's family.

In my family the pattern is different—on my father's side a history of blame and revenge and the men of the family having quick, violent tempers. On my mother's side, the pattern is one of bearing grudges for generations. So when I mapped out my family tree of forgiveness, I realized that on one side I had rage and anger and revenge and on the other the bearing of a lifelong grudge. Quite a combination!

Tina comes from a big farming family in Scotland. In many agricultural families, land can be the source of the family narrative of forgiveness. *"I think there were a lot of hurts held on to for generations and certainly I know my father was never able to forgive his father for the way that he perceived his father had treated him."*

Tina's father didn't inherit the family farm and land until he was fifty, when his own father died. He resented waiting so long for what was rightfully his. *"He had no capacity in his heart to understand why his father might have behaved the way he did toward him. It had an impact on everything that my father did ever since. It was paramount in our lives; it was one of the main playlists in our family."*

Although Tina was handed this narrative of forgiveness, it never seemed quite right to her, perhaps because she could instinctively feel the damage it was doing to the family and would continue to do if left unaddressed in her own life.

In fact the grudge has been passed down the family line to the next generation. The father tried to change the family map by handing the land to Tina's brothers early, before his death. So there was a huge willingness to change the story. Sadly, the issue of forgiveness was never looked at. Now the father is angry that his own sons are not grateful for not having to wait to inherit the land. So the grudge has mutated but been handed on nonetheless. As though the ability to bear a grudge was part of the inheritance.

"Unfortunately the pattern of his grudges hasn't changed in the next generation. My father resents some of his own sons in the same way and there's the same repeated pattern of enmity between my father and particularly my youngest brother and they hardly talk."

When your map is finished, take a good look at it. See if you can come up with a few words to sum up the major elements. In my case it was grudge and revenge. Sue just had a series of question marks; Linda thought *"isolate," "blame," "cast out," "low self-worth."* These are the words you have been given to navigate with—the headlights on your forgiveness car. Not very helpful, are they?

The good news is that it can all change. Your family narrative is just your family's accepted way of telling the forgiveness story. If you are mapmaking in a group, it's really helpful to compare notes at this point—you will be astonished at the different themes that come up. They will help you to understand that these stories are just stories: everyone has a different one. They are not the truth; they are not set in stone. Now you have all decided to tell a new story, free from the limitations of the past.

Becoming aware of your map, seeing it written down on paper is the first step to positive change. You might want to write your stories down and how you felt about discovering your family's narrative. Also put the key words and themes into your notebook.

Now it's time to destroy the map—take another good look at it—then tear it into little pieces or burn it, but make sure that you physically destroy it. Many people feel reluctant to do this. After all, even if it is not a very good map, it's been given to you as your main navigational tool by your family. At least it is a map. How are you going to navigate the waters of forgiveness without one?

What we are going to do is draw a new map. But you need to destroy the old one first. And as you do, remember that it actually wasn't a very good map; it didn't get you to where you needed to be. The best that can be said for it is that it has got you to this point, right here and right now, ready to destroy it.

Time for a new map

Now we are going to make a start on the new map. You are going to make two lists: one I call the easy list and one the hard list. Hard list first—on this list I want you to put the people who have done you a great wrong, or the ones who you are struggling hardest to forgive. Most people put parents, siblings, past relationships, and partners on this list. The hard list is made up of names that spring to mind right away when we begin to think about forgiveness.

The easy list is anyone who has ever done you a minor wrong, from the person who bumped into you at the supermarket, to the kid who pulled your hair at elementary school. Make sure the list is as comprehensive as possible; a list of all the people in your life you need to forgive. It doesn't matter how long it is, or how small what you need to forgive them for. . . . make sure that you leave no one out.

Don't worry if you can't think of many people to put on your map at first. They will come thick and fast once you start thinking about it. You may find it helpful to divide the list up into different areas: "Family" "School" "Work." Don't be afraid at how long the lists are either—this is the accumulated forgiveness luggage of a lifetime—I had about a hundred people on my original easy list. I was shocked at how, once I started remembering, I could recall the boy who had pulled my braids in elementary school, the woman who had pushed in front of me on the subway a month before, the hairdresser who'd made me look terrible when I was a teenager. Get them all down!

Everyone says that forgiveness is a lovely idea until he has something to forgive.

C.S. Lewis

Sometimes the idea of starting the lists can be frightening. It shows us in black and white just how far we have to go. It's like a declaration of willingness to start on this journey that we have avoided for so long.

Chloe, whose family tree was covered in grudges, was so scared that, initially, she couldn't come up with a list at all. *"I couldn't think of anyone to start with, but I did in the end find a few main areas for the easy list, when you start thinking about all the people in different parts of your life. I ended up with a very long list!"*

What about yourself, the navigator? Most people forget to put themselves on the list. We are often so busy concentrating on what the rest of the world has done to us that we forget that forgiving ourselves is central to the process. In fact you may want to put yourself on both lists! You can read more in Chapter 4 about learning to forgive yourself. Put these lists aside for a moment and concentrate on a new list. You may find this list uncomfortable—write down all the people from whom you need to ask forgiveness. Again make up an easy list and a hard list. Take your time; is there anyone you have left out?

As you are writing people down on the lists, notice the feelings that come up with their name. You may be surprised at how strong your reactions are, even with some people on the easy list. Notice the feelings—you may even like to make a quick note about them—but don't dwell on them at this point. Keep making the lists.

Time to put the baggage down

Think about when you last traveled and packed too much luggage—remember how difficult it was to carry to the station or airport, how you wished you had packed less stuff? Remember how your shoulders and arms ached with the weight of your cases and how grateful you were to put them down, what a relief it was to get to your destination and not have to carry them any more?

Your forgiveness suitcases are just the same. You may not be conscious of carrying them alongside you in life, but they weigh you down just the same. Imagine letting go of the burden of those cases; how much easier your life journey would be. Each person who appears in your lists is like an obstacle on the smooth path of your life. Imagine how much easier it would be to live your life, to forge ahead without all these people to trip over. Every single one of us has a few people on the list who are more than minor obstacles: they are the people with whom we have serious forgiveness issues. Not so much obstacles as heavy suitcases we trail alongside us.

Sometimes we don't realize what a burden our cases are until we let them go. Clare had a dream that made her laugh when she woke up, it was so obvious what she needed to do with her forgiveness cases.

"I was at an oasis in the desert; it was green and shady and beautiful. Behind me was a whole stack of luggage, all sorts of cases and trunks. I wasn't worried about them, just aware that they were there and I needed to keep my eye on them. I went to the edge of the water and had a long cool drink. I looked up and in the haze of the distance, I saw what looked like a camel train coming in my direction. I watched it for what seemed like hours as it came toward the oasis. When it got to the oasis there were about thirty camels with some riders with them. They all had a drink and filled their water bottles; they must have been traveling for a long time, you could see how happy they were to find water.

Then the head man came over to me with a clipboard, asked me my name, and said he had come to take all the luggage away. I was surprised but it seemed like the right thing to do and one by one the cases and trunks were loaded on to the camels, till there was nothing left.

The head man made me sign for the cases, saluted me, and got on the camel. Slowly the camel train turned around to head back off into the desert and on the lead camel was a big sign 'The lay your burden down camel train.' They loped off into the distance and I was left on my own at the oasis with an immense feeling of freedom."

While your own forgiveness luggage may not be as obvious as Clare's, it will certainly be weighing you down.

- How often do you find yourself going over old arguments, or things that you can't forgive, in your mind?
- How often does the same issue of forgiveness come up with different people?

❧ Do you feel that you are going through the same unhappy relationships again and again?

Even more seriously, it may be that these issues are buried deep inside your heart. You may feel it would be too painful to look at them, that they are better left buried.

But that is where the heart constricts and begins to build protective layers around your pain that both stiffen your resolve not to change, and make it more difficult to access those areas of pain. So as the years go by and maybe something prompts you to remember the incident or the person who hurt you, you will find you have to go through deeper and deeper layers of protection to access the memories. But underneath the protection the pain is still as raw.

Over the coming weeks you will find that you add people to the list. That's fine. Spend some time looking at it and see if you can begin to see a pattern. Remember your themes from your old map— do any of them ring true with some of the people on your list?

It's important to make two lists, easy and hard, for those you need to forgive and also be forgiven by, because they need different treatment. Taking the easy list first, you are going to take these people one by one, bring them through the process of forgiveness, and then cross them off the list. Once they are crossed off they will disappear off your forgiveness radar for ever.

The hard list is different. You will still be involved with many of the people on your hard forgiveness list, and so forgiveness will be an ongoing issue with them. But it will be so much easier once you have realized what your core issues of forgiveness are. You will no longer just hear the family narrative and replay it, falling right into the trap of grudge or revenge or isolation or passive aggression.

With your new understanding of how the forgiveness process works, you will have enough distance not to have your buttons pressed immediately, so that you go into an instant learned response. Instead you will learn to say to yourself, "Interesting—here's someone who's pressed that old forgiveness button yet again—what am I going to do about it?" And as soon as you have that distance you will no longer be caught in your family's story, you will be telling your own story of forgiveness, using your own map to navigate with.

3

Forgiving the Past
and Letting It Go

Forgiveness is letting go of all hopes for a better past.

A Course in Miracles

OUR CORE ISSUES of forgiveness are like a motto we carry stamped on our hearts. They run right through our hearts. For one person it might be "victim," for another "martyr," for a third "needing to be listened to." But one thing is certain: we all have one or more core issues of forgiveness, that is, the underlying problems that need resolution.

It is often the most difficult experiences in our lives that engrave the lettering on our hearts. Somehow the dark times encapsulate our beliefs about the world, the way we expect people to treat us, the issues that make us really angry.

When you are able to forgive and let go of the past, your core issue will lose its power over you. It will always be there, like an old scar, because you can't erase what happened to you, but when you have brought it out into the open and resolved it, the lettering will be so faint that you will barely be able to make out the words. One day someone will do something that would have sent you into a red mist before and you will simply register it and deal with it. And probably find yourself smiling, as you recognize the fact that your core issue has lost the power it once had.

When you start working your way through the forgiveness lists, you may find your core issues surfacing more often than usual. Suddenly people at work, or in your family, will be driving you mad in a very specific way and you will find yourself extremely grumpy with them. It will seem as though people are trying to make your life difficult. As always, this has nothing to do with them! It is your spirit trying to bring the core issues to the surface for you to have another look at them.

If you have the courage to look these issues straight in the eye and see them for what they are, eventually their power to send you into a rage will fade. By using the step-by-step process outlined in Chapter 5 you will be able to confront your core issues and find forgiveness. First you might need some help isolating and identifying your own core issues.

Finding the trigger

You know you are dealing with a core issue when something apparently insignificant sends you into a rage. So just sit for a minute and remember the last time you felt really angry. Now ask yourself these questions:

- ❧ What happened the moment before you got angry?
- ❧ Was there a particular person involved?
- ❧ Did it remind you of anything?
- ❧ Have you felt angry about this before?
- ❧ Is this a situation that keeps happening in different ways

with different people?

Answering these questions honestly will lead you straight to your core issues. Still looking for clues? Does the same issue keep returning again and again with different people? Is there something that people (they may be friends, family, coworkers, or complete strangers) frequently do in your life that just makes you feel like yelling? Bingo! You've found your core issue.

This is the way our spirit has of asking us to look at the core issue again. Are we ready to really look at it and try to resolve it? It's hard work, because it means examining and probably changing our knee-jerk reactions that may have seemed to serve us well as protection or defense mechanisms up to now.

Let's take a look at some typical core issues.

Testing and trusting

I have two core issues: I need to be listened to and I need people to be reliable. Both are a result of the abduction. If someone had been willing to listen at the time, I might not have kept it a secret so long. Reliability is a key quality for me—if I needed you in a life-saving crisis, would you be there for me? So people who don't listen to me or to others enrage me. It is one of the reasons I became a journalist, to listen and allow others to tell their stories. It is why I am "a good listener" and hear the subtext in conversations that others seem to miss. It is particularly important to me to listen to children and I hate it when anyone doesn't listen to a child.

People who don't listen get short shrift with me. As do the unreliable. If you are late for an appointment with me, I'll give you fifteen minutes' grace and then you had better contact me on my cell phone or have a pretty good reason for being late. Or I am gone. I find that all my close friends are good listeners and reliable. When

I meet someone new who might become a friend, those are two of the qualities I look for. If they are not there, I mentally make a note and feel that the person will never be a close friend.

Choosing the wrong partner time after time

We all know people who choose the wrong partners. Some of them seem to have an uncanny ability to choose the same sort of wrong partner over and over again. His teeth fit her wounds and her teeth fit his. Yet they are often caught up in a very passionate relationship. Even if they do split up, they'll go on and choose a similar partner, even similar looking. How often have you been struck by a public figure's mistress being an uncanny younger lookalike for his wife?

What these couples are unconsciously doing is trying to resolve a core issue. Until they do, they will act out the same problem again and again with the new partner, who is a variant on the unsuitable.

Injustice

Chloe found it easier to cast offenders into the outer darkness rather than deal with the pain in her heart. *"I just couldn't let go. If I got hurt I just couldn't, I couldn't bear it. I don't like injustice, I think injustice was what always brought on a grudge in my mind. To me it seemed the grudge I had against them justified all the actions I was taking, from the moment the bad thing happened. For example, not wanting to see people anymore, anger, whatever emotions I was expressing were justified by the grudge, so it didn't get worked out. I just cut them off, got rid of them."*

Chloe found she just couldn't let go of the hurt, no matter how often the other person apologized or tried to do something to make things better. Once the offender had crossed some invisible line (that he or she probably hadn't even known existed), that was the end.

Family conflicts

No one can press our core issue buttons like our family. After all, they are our past and have had a lifetime of practice. Put two adult siblings with problems in a room and within the hour they will have reverted to the age they were at when they were most difficult with each other. No matter that one of them is now a captain of industry and the other a leading light in one of the caring professions. They will be at each other's throats in a way that outsiders would find impossible to understand. Pretty much every family gives rise to core issues—and it is also where the early patterns of forgiveness are played out. There are many variants on the family core issue and most of us will have at least one! Try some of these on for size:

- Absent parent
- Violent parent
- Drunk parent
- Not loved as much as the other children
- Scapegoat
- Too much responsibility (oldest sibling)
- Left out of things (middle child)
- Treated as baby (youngest)

Let's look at some common examples of core issues in families.

Being a victim

As a child Linda was constantly bullied by her two older brothers, with no protection from her parents. So although being a victim is a horrible place to be, when people treated Linda badly, it felt familiar, literally. Because her brothers were continually playing tricks on her, this has also affected her ability to believe in the genuine generosity of others. *"It makes it hard to receive and let people in—I keep thinking, Is there going to be a sting in the tail? Recently I had two men friends over for lunch at Easter—they arrived and handed me a warm thing wrapped in tissue paper. I said, "Is it a dead bird?" It was a painted egg."*

Linda says that everyone, including herself, was shocked by her reaction. What guest would wrap up a dead bird and bring it over as a gift? But that was exactly the sort of thing her brothers would have done and for a moment she was plunged straight back into childhood.

Until we deal with our core issues we are all like Linda, just waiting for our core buttons to be pressed, to be taken straight back to the difficult moments of our lives. It has nothing to do with what is really going on, but it is deeply hurtful and upsetting. And of course, the people who are inadvertently pressing our buttons often get a completely inappropriate reaction. They are in the present, whereas we are acting out a narrative that is long past but still haunts us because it is unresolved.

Anger

We all know angry people who can relive the tiniest detail of a conversation that may have happened years ago. They are caught in a web of anger, stuck there with the core issue. Generally the key that someone is getting close to one of your core issues is that sudden wave of uncontrollable anger that washes over you and probably has not very much to do with the person right in front of you—that person is just the messenger. Unfortunately, messengers are also often the ones who get shot. But don't worry, the messengers just keep coming until you get the message!

Because she is also a survivor with a strong personality, Linda's way of surviving this victim label, once she left home, was anger—sometimes shown appropriately, sometimes not. As Linda later recognized, the problem with free-floating anger is that the target is often paying for things that have nothing to do with him or her. So Linda would be buying a coffee in a bar and the server would say something in a slightly sarcastic tone that would remind Linda of her brothers. Linda was now determined to defend herself, not let anyone bully her like that again. So she would get out the flame-thrower. "*It was debilitating as well as helping me. I could only be myself by being angry and assertive.*"

This happens all the time in public, someone ranting at something that seems fairly inconsequential to the rest of us. But the person ranting has been plunged straight back to his or her core issue and if it hasn't been addressed, the only defense is attack. Haven't we all been there? Someone upsets us and we can't respond, for one reason or another. Perhaps the person is gone before we can think of the right response, or it's in front of other people we want to impress. So we get on the bus and the next person who treads on our psychological toes gets it in the neck.

Sibling rivalry

Chris comes from a big, close family. She is one of seven brothers and sisters and is expecting her first child next year. Chris is sandwiched between an older and a younger sister in the pecking order, and although she gets along well with the older Anne, there has often been tension with the younger Pat. "*I have to admit that between me and Pat there has always been a lot of competition, always. We were very close in age, and all through our teenage years Pat was the glamorous one, the attractive one.*"

When Chris found out she was pregnant, she was delighted and couldn't wait to tell her family, although she knew that Pat might be sensitive about the news, because she had just come out of a big break-up with a man she had hoped to marry.

Chris had planned to tell her sister on the way home but there was a mix-up at the train station and another brother turned up as well as Pat to meet Chris. *"I had by accident sent a text message to my brother instead of her, asking him to collect me even though I'd arranged it with her. She was very offended, over the top offended. I just didn't tell her I was pregnant, because she was in bad form and it was as much as I could do to get over having sent the wrong message to the wrong person. She seemed to think I'd done that to get at her."*

Chris told her mother the news first. *"I told my mother, largely because I just wanted to tell somebody. My mother was sworn to secrecy, she wasn't supposed to tell anybody but of course when we were all together and after a few drinks my mother announced it to the whole dinner table. My sister Pat was there, as well as some of my other brothers and sisters. Pat was really offended and right there and then walked out of the house and wouldn't come back and hasn't spoken to me since."*

Absent parents

Everyone has core issues. None of us is immune, even counselors. Joe runs a successful alternative therapy center in the west of England. There are various practitioners and he himself is a gifted counselor, with appointments booked weeks ahead. Former clients are full of praise for his sensitivity and their ability to trust him enough to dare to begin the long and difficult journey of change. He starts by laughing as he tells me his story, but pretty quickly astonishes both of us with how angry he feels.

"My parents never really listened and it seems to be a recurring theme in my life that I come up against people who don't listen and they drive me crazy. I get rid of them and then another one pops up. I was best man to someone like that and no sooner had I edged him out of my life than I took on someone at work who turns out to be like that too and it drives me mad."

Recently Joe has taken on another therapist in his center and is surprised to discover that exactly the same core issue is coming up with this new colleague. *"He doesn't listen and thinks he is really clever, just chatters on and drives everyone mad. I had to go out to dinner with him the other day and I managed not to fight with him during dinner, though I was pretty abrupt. But when I got home my wife had to scrape me off the ceiling and talk me down for ages, I was so angry."*

I had never heard Joe raise his voice about anything before now, but it was hard to stop him ranting about the new member of staff. He was really angry, reliving how painful the situation was for him.

Distance

Sometimes letting go of our core issues comes in the most difficult and painful circumstances. Tony grew up in a family where both his mom and dad worked, *"never really having time for the children."* He had a difficult relationship with his elder brother, who was six years older than him. They got into a lot of fights, which Tony, being younger, inevitably lost. *"I hated my mom and dad for always giving their work first priority and I hated my brother for not playing with me and beating me up instead. This dynamic has set some pretty harmful patterns in me. In my teens, my biggest dream was to become independent and leave the family."*

Tony was driven to be successful and independent but now finds that *"it also can make you very lonely."*

Meanwhile his brother had become a drug addict and there were a lot of problems in the family because his parents denied his using drugs and only wanted to appear to be the perfect family to the outside world.

Tony did the classic thing and cut himself off from his brother at the age of twenty-five.

"In my early thirties he and I did make some attempts to reconnect, but there was no basis of trust and too much hurt to have a continuing relationship."

Martyr

When Betty's father was ill during her childhood, her mother leaned on her and confided in her in a way that was a heavy burden for a child. It also meant that she saw at even closer hand than usual how her mother operated emotionally, saw the motto stamped on her heart; saw her core issues close up.

"My mother held grudges; she'd often assess people by the wrongs they'd done her years ago and she couldn't get past that. If they had done something that she deemed unjust or wrong she would always refer back to that, regardless of whether they had done a great deal since, such as look after her while she was ill or remember her birthday or whatever.

When I was a child, I remember once when she was unwell and she wanted me to stay with a relative. At the time the cousin was very busy and she just couldn't put me up for the night. That was years ago. Because of that, every time that cousin did something that my mother thought was selfish, she'd refer back to that incident. She'd never confront the person, never talk about it in front of them, and therefore she never felt in a position to forgive them because she kept going back to whatever it was."

Tina's mother was also something of a martyr and Tina recognizes that, not surprisingly, to some extent she has inherited the martyr core issue that her mother had. "I suppose my efforts, my energy, my contributions in a personal and professional capacity not being recognized and acknowledged would be an issue. If I feel that I am being taken for granted it fills me with resentment. I work hard and people don't recognize it. I invest a lot in my personal relationships and take great care with them and then I have to step back sometimes and say, 'You idiot, they didn't even think about you there. Why did you bother putting all your energy, your precious energy, there? It was ill used.' And that is hard to forgive because I can't believe that people can be so careless. It seems to me that I wouldn't be so careless, but then those are issues for me about expectations and about being a victim or a martyr."

Forgiveness does not change the past, but it does enlarge the future.

PAUL BOESE

Strategies for change

A time may come when you see this chance to identify your core issues and deal with them as a gift from the whole forgiveness process. By bringing them out into the world, the issues lose their ability to send you diving straight into the red mist, or depression, or grief, or whatever your reaction happens to be. Recognizing and naming your core issues allows you to deal with and resolve them. If we can learn to identify our core issues, we can forgive the past and let it go. There are several key strategies for letting go of your core issue.

Identifying the trigger

Once you can find out what triggers your core issues, you are more than halfway to resolving them. Make a list of the last five times you felt extremely angry or sad or depressed. Can you begin to see a pattern? Is there a certain situation or type of person who sets you off? Once you think you have identified the trigger, watch out for it the next time it appears and see how you react.

A sense of distance

Identifying the trigger gives you the chance to see the situation coming. At first, expect to be plunged right into the anger or sadness or depression as usual. But in time you will make the connections and will see the situation coming. Giving yourself a few seconds even to say, "Aha, this is familiar and usually makes me angry/sad/depressed," offers you the chance to react differently. Eventually you will see the situation coming and be able to sidestep it like a martial arts master.

This is your core issue and yours alone— it is up to you to deal with it

Your core issues are unresolved pain rooted in the past. To let go of them is to let go of the past that has formed you into who you are today—and that is hard. It can feel as though letting go of the past is letting go of your own identity—who would you be if you dared to be different? In that situation what we do is wait for the other person to change, to "give in" first. Forgiveness teaches us that we are the only people who can change. Because when we change, the whole nature of our relationships will change too.

Not blaming anyone else for how you react to your core issue now

Being aware of your core issues is the first step to doing something about them. Recognizing your core issues gives you enough distance to look at the message rather than shoot the messenger. People who press your particular core issue button often don't even know they're doing it. Eventually you may get the message and try to do something about it.

If this was not a core issue for you, how would you react?

It's always surprising to watch someone dive off the deep end when it's not your button being pressed. You can see that the person who is losing control is doing so completely out of proportion and out of context to what has been said. That's because the person is not reacting to the present situation at all, but to a very strong trigger from the past. We can see it in others, but it is really difficult to recognize it in our own reactions. Can you begin to imagine having the distance to say—"Look at that person pressing buttons for me?"

What would happen if you did it differently?

Imagine not reacting in the way you usually do. This may still be impossible in the real situation when you are being triggered to respond in oh-so-familiar ways. So it is worth visualizing situations you have been in the past and rewriting the script in your head. How could you have been different? What would have happened instead? Then next time you are feeling drawn into the same situation, remember that you have already rewritten the script once and try it out in real life. It may not work. But you are taking the important step of saying, "I can do this differently, the patterns are not set in stone."

Using the Strategies

I believe that God (or if you prefer, the universe) is always giving us another chance to resolve our core issues. The wonderful way we bump into them every day is surely about resolving or checking in on how we are doing with them. All the relationships we have, both casual and more complex, are ways of us all moving along in our emotional development.

Sometimes when I am having a good day, I can recognize a core issue person when he or she appears. The person who promised to do something for the reading group I belong to and "forgets," as she has a hundred times before. On a good day I will say to myself,

"Here is the unreliability issue again. How are you feeling about it/going to deal with it this time?" Of course on a bad day, I'll be ranting to her answering machine before I've even checked how it makes me feel.

Or someone at work will ask me a question and not listen to the answer. On a good day I will understand that the person is distracted because he or she is busy, and I'll wait for a quieter moment, then try again. On a bad day it will drive me to distraction.

Here are some examples of how you can employ the strategies outlined above to confront and resolve the core issues we looked at earlier.

Testing and trusting

I once worked on a complicated project with someone who was never really there in spirit. She didn't listen and was always running to catch up with herself. So she would ask a question and not listen to the answer, when I knew that listening would influence our work for the next week. Not listening meant that I often had to take up the slack, when if she had listened in the first place, we could have saved ourselves so much work.

It was incredibly hard for me to deal with until one day I visualized her as an immense button coming toward me with "I don't listen. What are you going to do about it?" stamped on her. It made me laugh and gave me just enough distance to realize that we had been thrown together so that we could both look at our issues. That I could choose to react differently rather than plunging into the abyss every time she asked me the same question for the third time. That I had turned up in her working life because I was a good listener, which gave her an opportunity to change.

I started sending her e-mails to deal with all her questions.

When she saw things written down, she somehow could take more notice. It also meant that we had a record of our communications, so that when things went wrong because she hadn't acted on the information, she would look back and see the e-mail marked urgent and be forced to take responsibility for not acting in time. It didn't resolve things completely, but it did enable us to work together without my feeling enraged for much of the day.

Choosing the wrong partner time after time

Because each new partner is a different version of the core issue that needs to be addressed (for example jealousy, violence, settling for less), in the end a person will come along who will be just different enough for you to want to change. Or some part of you will be ready enough for change so that the right person to lead you to that change will suddenly appear in your life. They may not be there for long, but their purpose is to lead you on to the first steps of the forgiveness path.

Injustice

Injustice was the lettering on Chloe's core issue and she needed to ask herself in what situation had she been a victim of injustice in the past that had made it so difficult to bear.

She has come to understand that the messenger of your core issue is just that—the bearer of a message that you should listen to. Forgiving the person and instead looking at the core issue he or she symbolizes may have long-term implications for the friendship. It may be that you need to end this particular relationship.

Chloe now has that essential distance between having her core issue button pressed and plunging into the red mist. *"What's changed is I'm more mature and at times like this I ask myself whether it is truly an injustice*

I'm smarting over? Maybe somebody is having a bad day or yes, there is a reason, they are saying something that needs looking at in me. It's realizing the truth that what I perceive as injustice often isn't."

Family conflicts

Sometimes when things change within a family, it takes time for us to catch up with how those changes affect our lettering and core issues. The more we have invested in hanging on to our core issues, the harder it is to accept change. But change comes anyway, whether we want it or not, and that can make our core issues resonate in an unbearably painful way. For if we don't deal with them, they don't go away but become rooted in us.

Being a victim

Linda has realized that her core issue is victimhood. This is well founded; she grew up the youngest in a family with two elder brothers who bullied her constantly without any protection from her parents. She was a victim. The problem is that she internalized this as a way of being in the world. *"When someone is hurting me, it feels very familiar. I don't know what it feels like to be intimate and not be a victim."*

Since Linda has recognized what her core issue is, the public fireworks have become less frequent. In the past she would have been in the middle of an argument before she realized what was going on. And mid-fight it is hard to go back, because you have already passed the point of no return when the adrenalin is pumping and the fight situation feels so familiar.

"I can let go more easily, but being a victim still feels bad and familiar. Someone was late to meet me recently and my immediate reaction was, 'That's typical.' Still being a victim."

By learning to trace her feelings of victimhood to the way her brothers made her feel as a bullied child, Linda is beginning to give herself the essential creative distance between having a core issue button pushed and overreacting. She may still get angry in a situation but she is beginning to have that "oh here I am again" feeling, which is the first step to acknowledging that this person who is making you so angry is really hurtling you straight back to another situation that made you angry. You'll eventually come to recognize that this person making you angry now shouldn't pay for the people who hurt you so much in the past, but is a chance to look at the anger and deal with it. *"The brothers still bubble up, but I don't feel the same panic. I also didn't realize how invested I was in being a victim, how that way of being is attractive to some other people."*

Working with forgiveness has given Linda the chance to tackle the core issue of her brothers' cruelty. She has been surprised to discover that they too were victims, in a different way. *"I don't mean that what they did was understandable, but it was not from a place of choice on their part, that makes a difference."*

Linda has worked hard not to see herself as a victim in her relationships and though she describes major changes in the way she deals with the world, she sometimes still has difficulties recognizing how much she has changed. *"I believe I'm ineffective, so I can't see the change in relationships. But I'm better at recognizing the situation and leaving before it gets too bad. By not going in as deep, I can get out sooner."*

Sibling rivalry

To an outsider the story of Pat's reaction to her sister's news of pregnancy seems extreme. Rather than being happy, she takes umbrage and refuses to speak to her. There is clearly more going on here. Sometimes it is difficult to unravel what the real narrative of a quarrel is, but if we think that every relationship we have is meant to give us a chance to resolve our core issues, or at least address them, we begin to have some indications of what might be going on.

Until now Pat's role in the family has been the attractive and glamorous one. The motto stamped on her heart might read "prettiest and most attractive to men." She might have expected to marry and have children before Chris. Now, not only has she split up from the man she was hoping to marry, but her sister—the one who didn't have "prettiest and most attractive to men" stamped out as her heart motto—has upstaged her, and without even bothering to let her know first. When you look at it from Pat's point of view, you can see why she might feel resentful—Chris has touched on Pat's most sensitive core issue. That of course doesn't excuse the clumsy and ungracious way she behaved, but our core issues, particularly when it comes to the family, can send us into another world in a nanosecond. It's more like a dream state than reality; the normal ways of behaving, or the ways we would even expect ourselves to behave, simply don't apply.

The other strange thing about core issues is how fixed our identifying labels become. Both sides accept the labels; both sides get ready to do that old familiar dance once more. It's as though the band strikes up and everyone accepts that this is the way that it has to be danced, each with his or her allotted partner.

So although Chris is hurt at her sister's reaction, she still feels a bit guilty. *"She was grumpy and behaved badly but I should have told her, and I do feel a little bit that I need to be forgiven."* As though she needs to take responsibility for her sister's lack of generosity. Pat can't bear to have the attention for "most feminine sister" taken away from her (and what could symbolize femininity more than pregnancy?).

Chris recognizes this too. *"I know there is more going on in this situation. I never heard what the other reasons were, though she clearly has a reason. She kept saying to people, 'Ask her, Chris knows, she knows what she's done, she knows what* the problem is.' I do know that I knew more about this man probably than anybody else did and knew how up and down it had been and how much her hopes for the future, her own hopes for having children, were vested in him.

I think she felt that I put her in a funny spot instead of warning her, knowing that she was sensitive and knowing that she would be upset. I think she thought that I set her up to be embarrassed or set her up to be hurt in front of my parents. She was always going to feel ambivalent about my being pregnant."

Distance

Tony had very little contact with his brother. Then he heard from a common acquaintance that his brother was suicidal. "My world was shaken again and I did not want to accept responsibility for this secret, so I told him to go and talk to my parents. My parents kept me out of the story, as I had long ago made clear that I had my own life to live and did not want to get involved in the drama of my brother all the time. My father basically tried to save my brother in the last year of his life and tried to get him back on track again, still trying to get him back to mainstream society and a paid job."

Tony went to see a counselor and explained the situation. "His advice was to say goodbye to my brother and release myself from him and so I did. I spent three hours with my brother in which he mainly talked about his life, about his experiences, our parents. He told me he had not been a very nice brother for me and I could see he was sorry. For me this saying goodbye was a way of protecting myself. When I left his apartment at two in the morning, he insisted on walking down the stairs with me 'to put out the garbage.' When it was time to say goodbye, he told me he loved me. I felt almost paralyzed and said in an automatic manner:'I love you, too' and got into my car and drove home."

Six months later he was watching an episode of the UK television series The Bible. "It was about Joseph being sold by his brothers as a slave. By the time his brothers came to Egypt and asked Joseph (by that time a very famous man) for food, I was crying out loud. I thought, If my brother knocks on my door now I will let him in and give him shelter. The whole issue about Joseph forgiving his brothers who had sold him made me cry and I did not know why. I have a strong belief this situation was given to me by God to prepare me for the things which were going to happen.

A week later we heard from the police that my brother was dead. In the last week of his life he had been writing poems and a letter in which he asked for forgiveness and he said he also forgave us."

Tony says that the death of his brother has totally changed his view of life. "I have become so much more conscious of God and the softer qualities that are important in our interactions and relationships, as before I was very business oriented."

If you think forgiveness is easy or for the weak ones, you have not tried it yet.

TONY

Tony came to realize that forgiveness was key to resolving the core issues with his brother and parents. He has let his brother go and come to a more peaceful understanding with his parents, though it has taken him some years and a lot of painful soul-searching. But he is sure that forgiveness is the key. "If we don't forgive we stay imprisoned by old fears, create more wounds out of old ones, and pass the hatred on to our children and they onto theirs without knowing why this all started. It has now become possible for me to heal instead of hate. I have also learned that if you don't forgive completely, if you keep that one handle just for security, you have not forgiven at all."

Martyr

We get many chances to look at our core issues. Feeling hard done by is a classic core issue for many women, turning from victim into martyr. When Betty's mother knew she was dying, she still found it hard to change.

"It was difficult. You'd think knowing she was dying would have made a difference. But because it was an attitude and a way of behaving that she had developed over sixty years and was so ingrained in her, actually it wasn't easy to change. You'd think that death would help people to think and change their ways but it doesn't always."

The death of a close relative or friend is often a time of reassessment of our core issues. Since death shakes our world, it shakes all the narratives we have taken for granted and often there is a feeling of seeing more clearly than usual. It can be an extraordinary opportunity for looking at what works for us and what has been accepted as a narrative in a way that is not particularly helpful. In this way the death of someone close, although extremely painful, can also be a strange liberation.

Since her mother's death the way Betty looks at life has changed too.

"I suspect I followed certain patterns of hers in the past, which could be summed up as martyrdom. If someone has done something bad to you, it's satisfying if you have the moral high ground. Of course you always maintain that upper ground, while you don't confront them, and they may have very justifiable reasons as to why they did it, but as long as you don't tell them how aggrieved you're feeling, you can feel very happy. So since she has died, I think I am probably better at exploring why I will sulk about things and I think I am getting better at forgiving."

Tina, who has inherited a strong martyr core issue from her mother, has taken the important step of recognizing that we are all responsible for teaching people how to treat us. Ask yourself, why do some people get taken for granted and others don't? Because we have taught people that if they treat us a certain way—well or badly—we respond. *"Life is reciprocal but I'm responsible for what happens, so it's more a question of what am I doing in those relationships that is causing this to recur that is important really.*

I'm working on creating the distance, the space to be objective, so that I can use my intelligence more effectively rather than react. In general, up until now I react, but I might not react immediately when it is healthy. I can't sometimes do that when people are taking advantage of me. I might be aware that they are but I don't do it immediately and then it builds up and there is a whole series of resentments that I seem to then blast out and I become in their eyes unreasonable, because it is so out of the blue. It's the last straw, because I haven't that more healthy conditioning to be able to immediately say when something is not right or good or fair to me, to be able to find what it is I need."

Using forgiveness as a tool for confronting your core issues

So can we ever get rid of that lettering running right through the heart of our forgiveness issues? Our core issues are there for a reason. They are there to bring us right up against our forgiveness issues, the themes we find hardest to wrestle with. The first stage is to recognize and acknowledge them. Then, we begin to understand that when people turn up in our lives and relationships and start pressing our core issue buttons, these are a wonderful opportunity to change our narrative. An opportunity to put some creative distance between us and the core issue so that we are not plunged into the difficult feelings straight away. Making other people pay for our previous hurts never works in the long run; it just makes us feel more guilty and isolated.

In my first month of looking at my own core issues of reliability and people who didn't listen, it seemed to me that everyone I met—on the bus, in the street, at work—was a shining example of someone who either didn't listen or was completely unreliable. In fact, one day it happened so often that I ended up laughing—and finally getting the message.

This was my issue: even though people were queuing up in the street to get me to practice, I could change things. So what if occasionally someone didn't listen to what I said? What was I, the Delphic oracle? Once I started being able to laugh at myself, I realized that sometimes it might not matter if someone asked me directions in the street and didn't listen to my answer. So what if they got lost?

So the good news is that the motto stamped on your heart can and will fade. I still need people to listen for the important stuff, but I have learned to ask for what I need (teach people how to treat you) so I say, "It's really important that you listen to this." And to my surprise, people usually do. Reliability is still important to me, but I don't expect people who are unreliable to change. I just don't ask them to do things that need reliability. They can still make me angry if they catch me unawares but I have learned that it is rarely life threatening. And I am thankful that my core issues have made me reliable and a good listener for others.

Spotting core issues in others

This is a very helpful exercise in understanding that we all have core issues and that we are bumping up against each other all the time. Why does someone irritate you so much? Why do you get someone else's goat just by walking into a room? Core issues . . .

Spend today making a mental note of the core issues of the people you come across. From the bus conductor, to the woman you buy your sandwich from, to the people you work with. Treat it as a game and see how many people you can identify. Just make a quick mental note: it might be "martyr," "victim," "judge," "helpless," "always right."

Once you realize that we all have core issues, it may help you to identify your own, particularly if you see someone flying off the handle, or behaving defensively, or letting themselves be walked all over in a way that is all too familiar to you. You will understand how our spirit is trying to lead us all to deal with our issues by bringing them out into the open.

You will notice a change in your life as soon as you identify and start thinking about your core issues. You may initially find that even more people turn up in your everyday life to test you out. It is as though your spirit is saying, "Great! She has finally decided to look at this! Let's give her plenty of practice!" That is when you need courage to continue with the forgiveness process into new territory rather than sink back into the old familiar ways. Accepting that every way that we reacted to the world is now up for change and indeed must change if we are to make progress on our forgiveness journey is painful. It will seem as though all the old certainties have gone with nothing to replace them. But it is the only way forward and it will get easier. Remember that you are drawing a new map and navigating through uncharted waters. It takes a little time to get used to the new geography.

Identifying these old patterns will likely churn up feelings of unease about yourself. But give yourself a break! In the next chapter, we come to one of the most important aspects of the forgiveness process and one that is easily overlooked: the importance of forgiving yourself.

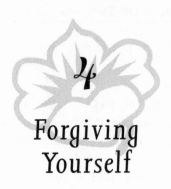

4

Forgiving Yourself

The supreme act of courage is that of forgiving ourselves. That which I was not but could have been. That which I would have done but did not do. Can I find the fortitude to remember in truth, to understand, to submit, to forgive and to be free to move on in time?

KAUFFMAN

*F*ORGIVING YOURSELF IS the final frontier. Most people find it easier to forgive almost anyone else. We are often harder on ourselves than on our worst enemies. Letting go of old grudges and grievances and long-held beliefs about ourselves is difficult. But the process is incomplete until you do.

Perhaps the most difficult part of the journey of forgiveness is facing ourselves. We can cut other people out of our lives; we can simply banish those people who have hurt us deeply. But we can't run away from ourselves or the voices that are nagging away in our head.

What forgiving yourself means

- You will stop beating yourself up for not being good enough.
- You will see yourself as precious in your own eyes.
- You will treat yourself as well and gently as the dearest person in your life.
- Those negative voices will lose their power.

Speedwriting exercise

Get a piece of paper and write at the top of the page:

Forgiving myself means . . .

Now spend three minutes just writing down a list of what comes to mind. Don't censor the list or try and think about it, just write. Now on the next page write at the top:

If I forgave myself, I would have to . . .

Now spend three more minutes writing a list, again without thinking about it too much. Read through what you have written. Are you surprised by it? When I did this exercise in a workshop some of the answers people came up with included:

Forgiving myself means . . .

letting my anger go
being free from unnecessary psychic violence
accepting my human frailty
not condoning my own bad behavior

If I forgave myself I would have to . . .

accept the deep truth of other people's nature
understand where I end and they begin
let go of an old self-image
accept that much of my life is beyond my control
accept that I am frail and human

Who do you think you are?

How did you ask yourself that question? Look at it again. Did you ask it in a tone of accusation or anger? Or as a simple question? The time has come to stop beating yourself up.

This is the key first step in forgiving yourself

The blame game

We all know people who berate themselves when little things go wrong in their day. Some of them seem to keep up a sort of running commentary of abuse at themselves: "I'm so stupid" . . . "oh, I'm hopeless at that" . . . "failed again." It's not hard to see how that can become the way a person feels about himself or herself.

Our internal dialogue—the background conversation we have with ourselves all the time—will often be a clear indication of how we judge ourselves. How often do these images come up in your internal dialogue?

- That was fantastic; you're really good at this.
- I wish I was as clever/pretty/funny as them.
- I should have done more exercise/work today.
- I shouldn't have had so much to eat/drink today.
- It's great just to be right here right now.
- I bet he/she/they don't like me.
- Why did they ignore me when they walked past?
- If only I could be more _____, I'd be happy.

Forgiving yourself is wrapped up in your own self-image—what were you taught about yourself when you were young? Sometimes our parents and teachers have inadvertently contributed to our low feelings of self-worth. When we did something bad they told us that *we* were bad, rather than what we had *done* was bad. If that is said to us often enough, we then internalize our parents' and teachers' beliefs about us and feel that we *are* bad.

Even if our parents didn't tell us that we were bad, they may still have given us messages about how little they felt they themselves were worth. We learn by watching—and those self-image narratives are transmitted down the generations.

Tina watched her mother beat herself up and it took her a long time to break free from that model. *"I'm better at forgiving myself than I was. I began to understand during my period of great crisis that part of the key was to try and forgive myself. It's difficult because I have inherited the tyranny of my mother; she's hugely tyrannical to herself. She was certainly extremely hard on herself, and I am hard on myself, but I'm trying to change that."*

You know you are beating yourself up when that familiar record starts playing in your head: "it'll never work" . . . "there's no point in trying" . . . "nobody loves me." Or when you hear someone else's voice berating you in your head—a parent or teacher who always managed to make you feel small and a failure.

Treating yourself as precious

Any process of forgiveness involves a change of heart. The world is no longer as we saw it. The people who hurt us lose their power to hold us stuck in that hurt. When we forgive ourselves, the change is even deeper and more powerful. Not only does our whole view of the world change, but the way we relate to the world inevitably moves on too. We change in such profound ways in relation to ourselves, that we no longer hear those painful voices of the past or give them any power over us.

Forgiving yourself means recognizing that you are precious. That there has never been and will never be anyone else like you in the whole universe.

An exercise in treating yourself well

Think of the people you love most in your life and a place where you have been happy together. It might be on vacation, or in a simple daily activity like making a cake, walking to school, having a laugh together. Do they know how much you love them? How? Think of all the things you would happily do for them to make them feel how much you care.

Now imagine yourself as a third person in that scenario—can you imagine treating yourself just as well as your most loved ones?

Take the same walk, bake the same cake, have the same laugh, except include yourself as a loved one in the scenario. How does it feel?

We need to treat ourselves as gently as the dearest person in our lives.

Forgive yourself for your faults and your mistakes and move on.

CONFUCIUS

You are allowed to get it wrong

We often find it hard to forgive ourselves because it is even harder to admit to ourselves that we got it wrong. But owning up—even if it is only to ourselves—can be a thoroughly liberating experience. We do get it wrong. So what? Who said we had to be perfect? Getting it wrong shows that we are human, we make mistakes too. It might even make us more understanding when other people get it wrong too (though don't bet on it!).

Let's be clear though—owning up is not the same as beating ourselves up. Owning up means coming clean about when we get it wrong. How would you describe yourself when you get it wrong?

- selfish
- insensitive
- unkind
- brutal
- violent

In the next section I will teach you how to forgive those who have hurt you. But before you master that technique you must be prepared to show yourself the same sense of mercy.

It's time to stop being so hard on yourself. Think of something you need to forgive yourself for. Now imagine your best friend coming and telling you he or she had done precisely that thing and wanted to forgive him- or herself, but was finding it hard. How would you feel about that? You would probably find it easier to help the friend let go of whatever it was. To explain that forgiveness is a journey and that your friend needed to step onto the path. So why don't you treat yourself at least as well as you would your best friend?

It's time to make some new lists—an easy and a hard list of all the things you need to forgive yourself for. It might help to describe certain character traits that you would like to change. Then work through them in the same way as you did with the other people on your lists. Keep this list by you to work through in the Forgiveness Room in Chapter 5.

Chloe has used the Forgiveness Formula successfully in many areas of her life but she has found it most difficult to apply to herself. She worked her way through her easy list of people to forgive and then began tackling the hard list. She felt she had grasped the essential elements of forgiveness and was happy to apply them in her life. But she admits that despite forgiving others who have done her serious wrong in her life, she has found it extremely difficult to forgive herself and that changing her attitude toward herself is still very much "work in progress."

"I'm very hard on myself. In the past, with myself, there was no room for any forgiveness. I'm very good at putting things off until tomorrow. Then sometimes, it's happened in my life, where it has really hurt, when there was no tomorrow to do anything about. When people died, for example, and that's when I got the hardest on myself."

Chloe smiles when she says, "*I'm better with myself now. I've started, but it will take time.*"

We all make choices in life that we come to regret. Tina found it hard to break free from her family narrative of self-punishment. "*For instance, I have had abortions. Sometimes through carelessness, I've ended up being pregnant when it felt wrong to be. I've been so angry with myself both for getting pregnant and because I had an abortion. I'm responsible for the decisions I made and the actions I took. I accept that, but I have been very angry with myself for being so stupid. I'm trying to be more gentle with myself.*"

Only those who have experienced forgiveness can truly forgive.

GEORGE SOARES-PRABHU

This is what the Canadian writer on forgiveness, John Monbourquette, calls "compassionate acceptance of ourselves." He also points out that people who are incapable of letting themselves be loved or of realizing that they are loved, are unable to love others. It is the same with forgiveness. If you cannot forgive yourself, how can you truly forgive others?

We are good at putting ourselves at the bottom of the list when it comes to forgiveness. For Tony, who always had difficulties with a brother who subsequently died of a drug overdose, it took a long time to change and forgive himself.

"*Because we had such a bad relationship, my brother dying was also a liberation for me—an era of worries, manipulation, and sorrow was over. I did a lot of work on this and yes, I had a lot of feelings of guilt, also connected to not really missing him when he died or being sorry for that. I can say I have forgiven myself completely. But* before doing so I had to go through all the things I had done wrong, and acknowledging to myself that I had also done things wrong was the hardest part of it. I had to become vulnerable, something I had never learned to do."

The hard list

The photo exercise

Find a photograph of yourself at the time you most need to forgive yourself. Study it closely. Do you recognize yourself? How were you feeling when the photo was taken? What is it you need to forgive in that person? Keep the photo on your fridge door or on your desk so that you see it all the time until you have come to forgiveness.

There will be events in our lives where we feel we have done something that is unforgivable. We may never have told anyone else. But there is a voice inside us that will not let it go. You need to be gentle with yourself.

The death of a child is a terrible tragedy for any family. For Denise Green it was made worse, as for many other families, by the discovery that her son William's body had been stripped of various parts after his death in the Alder Hey Hospital in Liverpool, UK. William was born in 1992 with a heart disorder but was never seriously ill. He became an outpatient at Alder Hey Hospital and when he was eighteen months old the consultant suggested an operation to correct the condition. The operation had a high success rate and William was healthy and growing so they decided to go ahead. The operation was on Valentine's Day 1994, and was a success but then ten minutes later William had a heart attack and died. "It was a terrible shock because no one expected him to die."

When a disaster like the death of a child happens, many parents blame themselves. It is the classic "what if I had done this or not done that"—a scenario that is a recognized part of the grieving process. For Denise the "what if" scenario was all the more unbearable and poignant.

"The worst memory was that when he died, I had been the last one to see him. He put up a fight in my arms during the anesthetic, said, 'Stop it, stop it.' I had to force the mask over his face. For a split second I thought, 'What are you doing? Grab him and run out.'

Of course when he died a few days later, I felt I should have listened. He could have been alive if I had pulled away . . . I knew in my heart I was a good parent . . . It was a terrible thought and I had to pray and ask God to help me."

Denise was not responsible for her son dying. It was a tragic accident. No one could blame Denise for what happened—except herself. When they discovered that his body parts had been removed without their permission it was even more difficult for Denise not to shoulder the blame. Letting go of William meant that she had to find a way to forgive herself—or carry that sense of blame on with her through her life. Denise felt she needed to find a way of explaining to William what had happened and asking for forgiveness.

"Years later I took an English course and we had to write an essay to someone who had died and I thought, I'll write a letter to William, and I imagined it going directly to him and him opening it. I told him of my feelings, that I was the last one with him . . . explained as though he could hear how much we loved him, the pain of the decision to let them go ahead with the operation. I told him what the doctors had said; that there was a 98 percent success rate. Then I said, 'My worst memory was holding you and you wanting me to stop' . . . and I asked him to forgive me."

When Luke was in his early twenties, he began to come to terms with the fact that he had been repeatedly sexually abused by a teacher while he was in elementary school.

"I hit a point in my early twenties where I realized that I wasn't fully alive, that my view on the world and on my own life was not as others saw it and that they were bearing fruit and reaping harvests in their lives that I wasn't beginning to reap or bear and I wanted to. I began to see how the abuse had clouded or had a profound effect on my perception of myself and the world around me, and due to that my self-esteem was very, very low."

When we come to this point, it takes a lot of courage to go to those dark places and discover why our world doesn't make sense anymore. Although he had been abused as a child, Luke was surprised to discover that there was a place where he needed to forgive himself for the consequences of that abuse.

"I hit a place in my grieving of realizing that I needed to forgive myself for not allowing that child the freedom to dance, to sing, to be creative. I'd crushed him, or rather he'd been crushed—that is the truth—and I'd never since allowed him to dance, which is very understandable and in no way my fault. However, there was an opportunity for that child to dance within me and I had to recognize that."

When I forgave the man who abducted me, I was surprised to discover that I blamed myself for letting it happen. Even though I was only eleven, it must somehow have been my fault—for getting in the car in the first place, for letting him drive off, for not telling anyone afterward. It was a long time before I realized that this was another direct result of the abduction: he had said I would go to prison if I told anyone, and I had believed him.

Then I realized that the forgiveness issues raised by the abduction were complicated. Not only had I blamed myself as an eleven-year-old, but my adult self also blamed her. I realized that it wasn't the adult me that I had to forgive but the eleven-year-old. And I had to reassure her that she would never be in danger again. That the adult Kathleen would always be there to look after her.

Some part of me was still the child, fearful and deeply mistrustful. I realized that since then I had always been on my guard, always divided people into those I could trust in a crisis (would they save me from murder if it came to that?) and those I couldn't. Friends had to prove themselves before I trusted them, and if they ever broke that trust, I cast them out into the outer darkness—not to feel safe with them was unbearable.

Having forgiven myself, I now don't automatically assume that people are untrustworthy until they prove otherwise. My guard is down. But I have been surprised to find that most people I meet are pretty trustworthy. That is not to say they are going to become best friends, but neither does it mean that they are going to seek to harm me.

We may also need to forgive ourselves for the path not taken. Throughout our lives, we will be faced with choices and it can seem that we went down the wrong road. But a life peppered with "if onlys" and "what ifs" fails to recognize that if you look back on the path you did choose to take, it has led you to where you are right now, which is absolutely the right place for you to be. Imagine that you are making a journey from New York to London. What would be the best route? Is there only one path? Our life journey is like that route—we may choose different paths, but they all lead us absolutely where we need to go.

It may have taken you five years to escape from an abusive relationship—so what? You have learned an invaluable life lesson there and won't need to walk that path again. Or you went for one career and realized that it wasn't for you and yet had the courage to start again with your real heart's desire.

We all make mistakes—that is what makes us human. So give yourself permission to get things wrong now and then. Resolve not to be harder on yourself than you are on others. Treat yourself at least as well as you would treat your best friend. The only mistake we can make is not learning from our mistakes.

PART

2

The Forgiveness
Formula

5

The Forgiveness Room

*I*N PART ONE, The Forgiveness Path, we looked at the reasons for engaging with the forgiveness process and some of the issues that might come up for you. In this section you will learn the practical tools of forgiveness, the keys to profound change. To begin the process of forgiveness, we are going to imagine a room deep within your heart: A room that has been closed and locked for many years and that we are now going to open to the light of forgiveness. A room that contains all the bitterness and sadness of not forgiving—and that has meant that there is a place in your heart that is stiff and cold. We are going to open up the room, spring-clean it, and make it a part of yourself again, so that no part of your heart is shut down. You are going to have complete control of the process and can stop or slow down whenever you want.

The Forgiveness Paradox

**Forgiveness is never about them, it's about you.
But what they did to hurt you may have nothing
to do with you at all.**

Understanding this is key to your journey of forgiveness. It is the hardest paradox to grasp. People hurt you for all sorts of reasons:

- ❧ accidentally
- ❧ because you were in the way
- ❧ because you reminded them of someone in their past
- ❧ because they hurt so badly they had to hurt someone else
- ❧ for no good reason at all

Whatever happened to you, it is your choice and your choice alone to forgive. It's got nothing to do with them at all (although a full confession on the *Ten O'Clock News* might help!).

Remember the Forgiveness Formula that underpins the whole book; it describes exactly what forgiveness does and does not mean:

- ❧ It means completely letting go of the hurt this person has done you.
- ❧ It means letting go of the hold this narrative has had on your life.
- ❧ It means getting rid of a piece of baggage that you will no longer have to carry around with you.
- ❧ It does not mean forgetting what has been done to you.
- ❧ It does not mean that you do not learn lessons from what happened to you.

Getting Started: The Toolkit

The Forgiveness Room is a powerful visualization technique that can yield great results if you are prepared to really engage with it. You may want to do this completely on your own or you may want to do it in a small group. In either case some of the ideas below may help you engage with the process.

Keeping a forgiveness journal

Buy yourself a notebook that will become your forgiveness journal. Write down what you hope to get from the process and how you hope to have changed by the end of this book. This is a private journal and you should keep it in a place only you have access to, so that you will feel completely free in writing.

Get into the habit of spending half an hour a day jotting down how you are feeling about forgiveness. You will be surprised as you begin to engage with the process how much your feelings will change and it will be enormously helpful to be able to look back as you move into different themes.

It will help you to integrate the Forgiveness Room into your life if you record your feelings at the end of each session—write down how it felt to be there and anything important that came up.

Dream diary

It can be very helpful to keep a dream diary, especially once you really start using the Forgiveness Room. Get into the habit just before you go to sleep of asking yourself a question that you are struggling with. A typical question might be

- Why does this person make me so angry/anxious/sad?
- What can I do about this situation at work?
- How can I deal with this particular difficulty in this friendship?

Keep pen and paper by your bedside and jot down any dreams you have. You'll find that you soon get used to writing down your dreams and going straight back to sleep. Soon you will find how much you can learn from your dreams, how they bypass your conscious mind to give you clear pointers to the answer to your question.

If you are doing this on your own, *take your time*. Remember how long you have taken to get here: there is no rush to get through the forgiveness process. It will take you through some difficult moments and you need to deal with yourself very gently. Be patient, take it slowly, and the journey will take on its own momentum. You will be surprised when you look back through the journal as you go through the forgiveness process. Feelings will change, old hurts will be healed, and bitterness left behind. Be brutally honest in the diary and keep it in a safe place where no one else can read it.

Meditation

Whether you follow the Forgiveness Formula on your own or in a group, there are two exercises that are crucial to the journey. Begin each session of work with ten minutes of meditation. It will help to center your spirit and leave the daily anxieties of the world behind. If you have not done meditation before, sit quietly in a comfortable chair, eyes closed, with your feet flat on the floor. Take a few deep breaths and quiet your mind.

Just be conscious of your breathing in and out, in and out. Focus on the breath. When you are quiet, let what wants to arise come. Look at it gently, allow it to be. Sit with it. Examine your body, your heart, your mind, and your spirit. When something comes up, let it be. Breathe with it, in and out. If what comes up is painful, do not resist it but let it be, surround it with love and attention. Try to name it—fear, anger, hatred . . .

Don't worry if you get distracted and your mind races to all sorts of subjects. Just bring yourself back quietly to the center again. When you have done enough, sit quietly for a while longer and feel the peace. Then open your eyes again, breathe deeply, and stretch.

You can also do silent walking meditation. Walk in a park or on the beach, not talking to anyone, just concentrating on your breath. Pain that has been kept tight within you will not vanish overnight, but you will be surprised how effective regular meditation will be.

Life breaths

The second crucial exercise is learning about life breaths. Before you start and when you finish each exercise, take five life breaths. Choose a word to describe your inner feelings right now—it might be "fear," "hate," "anger." Take a deep, slow breath in through your nose, breathing in the opposite word: "hope," "love," "peace." Now slowly and deeply, breathe out through your mouth, a good strong breath out, breathing out the fear—hate—anger—word.

Do this five times at the start and finish of every exercise or whenever the negative feelings seem too much for you. As you move further into the Forgiveness Room, you will find that the negative words will change: they may be stronger one day, weaker the next. Always do the exercise gently. Your life breaths will help you change.

Working in a group

Many people find that the forgiveness process works better in a group. You can see that other people struggle with issues just as they see you struggle with your difficulties and that can be a great comfort. Doing the work in a group also makes sure that you do your homework and show up for this difficult journey!

If you decide to approach the Forgiveness Formula in a group, you may find that an odd number of people is most helpful—three or five, so that you don't pair up. Choose people you trust, with whom you have no major issues of forgiveness. Agree that you will meet once every two weeks at the same time, in a place that is quiet and confidential—no partners or children. Take the exercises slowly and only move ahead when you are all ready.

Most importantly, agree that whatever is said in the room stays in the room—it is never discussed with anyone else.

During each two weeks, do each exercise at home on your own and then bring it to the group. Make it a rule to write down what comes up for you and to read it to the other members of the group in turn.

Learning to listen

You need to feel completely safe to engage with the process of forgiveness. If you don't feel safe, you won't be able to address some of the deeper and more painful issues that will come up. The most important rule for the group is active listening—this means that when one of the group is talking, the others listen. No commenting, no judging, no opinions, just active, respectful listening.

For many of you this will be the first time you have talked about these issues, and comments from other people are not helpful. Offering comments or suggestions for change interferes with the process. Your journey is your own and if the group intervenes then it becomes something else. Your journey needs to be witnessed by the group but it is your journey and yours alone.

Listening buddy

Many people find it helpful to have a listening buddy through this process. You pick someone from the group and you either meet or talk on the phone once a week. You might like to go for a walk in the park or along the beach. You take it in turns to talk for five or ten minutes with no interruptions. The other person simply listens and makes sympathetic noises. It is an immensely powerful exercise that will help you to articulate what is really going on. Again, both of you will need to agree that these conversations are completely confidential.

Equal time

When the group meets, make sure that you all have equal time to speak—have a clock handy and time five or ten minutes each.

Appoint one person timekeeper for the evening and get them to ring a bell (or a spoon against metal!) at the beginning and end of each time limit. You can always come back for another five or ten minutes each when everyone has spoken. The important thing to get used to in a group is having equal time. Some people are better at talking in groups than others and if you don't time each other, they will naturally, if inadvertently, speak more than others. Even if you just sit in silence during your allotted time and feel unable to speak at first, it is important that it is still your time and that this is respected by the group.

For many of you this will be the first time that you háve looked at forgiveness, and it needs supportive silence to be heard. You may want to spend the first session together in a group talking about your arrangements and the ground rules for the group. It's important that you stick to the meeting times where humanly possible.

You may want to take a break in the middle of the evening and have something to eat together. But you should make it a rule not to discuss in detail what has come up during the session. It may be helpful to talk about something else entirely or how you are finding the process, whether you are giving yourselves enough time, when you find the best time of day is, whether you found one exercise particularly hard.

When you meet, it's a good idea to start the group by doing ten minutes of quiet meditation so that you can leave all the anxieties of the outside world behind. Follow this by the life breath exercise. Then each of you should check in for five minutes and say how the preceding two weeks has been for you. End the evening with five minutes each on how the evening has gone for you and another five minutes of meditation, followed by five final life breaths.

Remember this is your process
and it takes the time it takes.

The Forgiveness Room

**The Forgiveness Room is central to the process.
Although it is an imaginary room, you will find the
metaphor a strong and powerful one.**

There are five stages to this part of the forgiveness process. You need
to feel comfortable with each stage before you move on to the next
one. It is vital that you proceed at your own speed: there are no
medals for getting there faster than anyone else! The Forgiveness
Room is where you are eventually going to bring people in order to
forgive and be forgiven, so it must feel completely safe, that it is 100
percent your space. To open up the Forgiveness Room takes courage.
Remind yourself that at each stage of the process you need only do
what you feel comfortable with. Indeed it is only when you feel completely comfortable and relaxed with one stage of the process that you
should go on to the next stage. Take as much time as you need.

Always find a quiet place to sit; inside or out in the yard, or a
favorite walk where you won't be disturbed for an hour or so.
Unplug the phone and tell your family not to disturb you—
although it's probably a good idea at this stage not to go into any
detail with them, or anyone else, about what you are doing. The
forgiveness process needs quiet and you will find it has a momentum all of its own. Being questioned about it all the time is not
helpful. The important thing is that you set aside a regular time,
probably at the same time of day, to visit the Forgiveness Room. It
may be ten minutes a day or an hour a week to start with. In this
way you will find a rhythm of your own.

As you go through the exercises, you will be surprised to find
that you want to go back to the room—you are even looking

forward to it, though what happens in the room may be painful. You are healing, and the heart and spirit love to heal. Once you have turned yourself in the direction of healing, your heart and soul will bring you back there joyfully.

Forgiveness is not easy, it is not to be undertaken lightly. You may find that you are not ready to forgive, or that other things come up for you when you use the Forgiveness Room. The important thing is to be gentle with yourself. If you are not quite ready, use the room as a test of how well you are doing. But above all take your time. After all, it has taken you a lifetime to get to the door of the Forgiveness Room; you can take several more weeks or months to feel comfortable there.

Let us begin the journey

There are five stages to this part of the forgiveness process: Opening the Door, Stepping Inside, Being Inside, Staying in the Room, and The Forgiveness List. When you feel comfortable with one section, then move on to the next part of the process. But each time you come to the Forgiveness Room, take time to go through all the stages again. So even though you may be far along the process, always take time to do the first four stages—Opening the Door, Stepping Inside, Being Inside, Staying in the Room—again carefully. You will find different things coming up as you get deeper along the path of forgiveness. They are a way of preparing your heart and spirit for the next part of the journey. If you are doing this in a group, it may be helpful to open the session, after you have done your meditation and life breaths, with a few sentences each on how things have changed in the two weeks since you last met. How have the four stages been different for you?

Although you may feel you want to rush through the different stages, take your time—the process of preparing your heart for forgiveness is as important as the forgiveness itself. To really forgive and let go of years of pain and bitterness takes time. If you are making this journey on your own, you may want to take several weeks or more for each stage. There is no correct cruising speed, only what feels right for you. Wait until you feel completely comfortable with how the door looks and feels, for example, before you go on to the next stage of stepping inside. This is not a race. Never skip a stage; and remember, you need to be gentle with yourself.

Whether you are making the forgiveness journey on your own or in a group, it is important that you write down your impressions for each stage. Over the two weeks between each stage, keep writing things down that occur to you. When you are further along the path, I suggest you still do the first four stages each time. Always write down a few sentences for each stage. You will be astonished at how different your responses are, depending on your mood and how difficult things have become.

No matter how hard any part of the Forgiveness Room seems, don't give up! If one stage is too painful, stay with it for a while and be gentle with yourself. If it seems impossible to move forward, give your heart longer to heal and go back a stage. Take your time. But stay with it. It may be that you need more meditation and life breaths; you may need to spend more time preparing the room. This is your Forgiveness Journey; you will make it sooner or later, but one thing is certain: you will go there. So there is no rush.

You are learning to treat yourself gently; give yourself time and open up to your innermost beliefs. This may be unfamiliar to you and when it gets difficult, you may feel like running away. Just do your breathing and meditation and take your time.

Make sure that you are comfortable with each stage before you move on to the next one. Some people go through the four stages quickly and then hit difficulties later. For others the very idea of opening the door to a place that has been closed for so long is scary.

Stage 1: Opening the Door

Do some life breaths and close your eyes. Each stage is best done with your eyes closed so you can listen to your inner voice. You're going to open the door to the Forgiveness Room. It's a door that has been closed, maybe even locked and bolted for many years. Take some time to look at the door. What is it made of? Is the wood dented and covered in cobwebs? What sort of doorknob is there? Does it have a big key? What color is the door? Run your hand down the wood: what does it feel like? Look at the door until it feels very familiar. When you are ready you are going to open the door. How does the thought of that feel? There is nothing to be afraid of. You can shut the door again whenever you like. In fact you might want to take a quick peek and slam the door hard! If you want to, spend the whole of this first session looking at the door, touching the wood, and maybe even dusting it down. Does it need a new coat of paint? Or a beautiful sign that you might like to make showing that it is the Forgiveness Room?

It took weeks for me to be able to even open the door. For a long while I just stood in front of it looking at the peeling paint, the quadruple bolts, the rusted hinges, the huge key, knowing that opening the door meant opening my heart to the possibility of forgiveness. That was a terrible struggle. I really didn't want to open a door that had so many bolts and locks on it and that had been shut so efficiently that no one could get in.

Yet a part of me also knew that I couldn't go back to the old life of holding onto my grudges. So I spent days just standing and looking at that door, until I knew every crack in it. Knowing that if I opened the Forgiveness Room, eventually I would have to look at the possibility of forgiving the man who had abducted me. For days and days in my head I would walk up the path to the door and just look at it and think, 'This is too hard.' But I kept coming back.

Then I thought the least I could do, since I was spending so much time here in front of the door, was to make it look a bit brighter. So in my mind I sanded it down, back to the original wood. I removed all the bolts and kept just one key. Then I painted the door a wonderful Mediterranean blue. I oiled the lock and hinges, took out the giant rusty key, and oiled and polished it.

So what does your door look like? Does it need redecorating? Take it slowly . . . be gentle with yourself. When you are ready turn the key, open the door. Notice how the door creaks on its hinges: it hasn't been opened for years. Push the door open as far as it will go. How do you feel? Stop whenever you want to. If at any point you have had enough, do your life breaths and stop. You can come back here whenever you want, as many times as you want, until you feel ready.

It was a relief for me to wrestle with the lock and bolts, listen to the door creaking on its hinges, and apply pints of WD-40 to make it open smoothly. Finally the day came; I was walking along a beach and looking at the waves breaking gently on the sand, feeling the warm water lap over my feet. I knew deep in my heart that I could do this, and in my mind I went up to the door as I had so many times before, admired the paintwork, turned the key in the lock, and opened the door. Then I put the key under a beautiful stone by the door. I never wanted to lock this door again.

Do your life breaths. Open your eyes. Spend a few moments sitting quietly, absorbing the feelings that have come up. Now write down your first impressions in your journal.

- How does it feel to have got to the door?
- What does the door look like?
- How far did you get in the process?
- How do you feel about what might be ahead?

Get in the habit of writing a few sentences or phrases each time you do the different stages—you will be surprised how your feelings will change over time. Watching the changes in your journal will help you to understand that you are on a journey.

Stage 2: Stepping Inside

When you are ready, open the door and step inside. Look around you. What does the room feel like? There has been no one inside here for years: is it cold and musty, damp and dark? Are there cobwebs hanging in the corners, plaster flaking off the wall, bits of rubbish on the floor? Take your time describing it and remember—you can leave any time you want to, closing the door behind you. You are in no danger; you are in total control and perfectly safe.

When I stepped inside my room, it looked as though someone had left in a hurry; there were cobwebs and dust and garbage. Boxes full of stuff sat in one corner, broken furniture in another. There was only the sunlight coming through the door to cut through the dusty gloom. The shutters on the windows were closed and it smelled musty, as though no light or air had penetrated this room for years.

I stood there, near the door, ready to run. Then I suddenly thought, This is what a room in your heart looks like. This is what you have been carrying inside you all this time. Is this how you want it to be?'

If it feels scary, leave the door open and stand just inside the room. Spend time just looking around the place, taking it all in . . . look at any furniture there might be in the room, boxes in a corner. This is the room of your heart that you have kept locked away and now you are going to reclaim it. When you leave you may want to lock up securely, or you may want to leave the door wide open or just a crack.

Before I left I opened the shutters and threw the windows open. The sunlight streamed in and I just stood there for a while, thinking, There is so much to do, but this might just be possible. Then I wedged the door open with a large stone and walked off down the path.

When you have finished, do your life breaths. Open your eyes. Spend a few moments sitting quietly, absorbing the feelings that have come up. Now write down your first impressions in your journal.

- ❧ How does it feel to step into the room?
- ❧ Can you describe what the room looks like?
- ❧ How do you feel about what you found in the room?
- ❧ Can you imagine staying in there—what would that feel like?

Stage 3: Being Inside

When you are ready, come back to the room. This is your space and you can let whatever you like happen there, because this is a virtual room in the imagination of your spirit. Open the door and windows and let the sun stream through. It's been a long time since there was any light or fresh air in the room. What does it feel like to let the sun in? Perhaps you would like the sea to lap gently against the door, or a good hard rain to fall outside to clear the air—imagine anything you like happening in and around your room that makes it feel safe and comfortable.

Everyone decorates the room differently—the important thing is that it is your room. You are going to spend a lot of time there and it's essential that you should feel comfortable there. So think about how you want to clean it up and make it yours. It doesn't have to stay the same—you can change it every time if you want to—you may need several tries to get it exactly right for you.

- What state is the room in now?
- How much stuff do you want to get rid of?
- What would make it feel like your room and completely safe?

Go with what springs to mind—if you need a moat, machine guns to protect you, and barbed wire round the door, that's fine too. Big bodyguards or bouncers guarding the path to stop unwelcome intruders—anyone or anything to make you feel safe.

For Laura, "It was like my kind of ideal room in a house would be and it was a source of comfort. It was absolutely lined with books from floor to ceiling and it had one wall that went out into this beautiful garden and big tables strewn with books. I suppose they represented huge, richer ideas and new opportunities and new ways of looking at things."

Chloe is a practicing Buddhist and her Forgiveness Room had a comforting familiarity. "It was just like my Buddhist center with lots of big bay windows, sunny with lots of air coming in and nature all around, very little furniture, minimalist."

Sue, a busy working mother with very little time or space to call her own, found it difficult to imagine a room at all to begin with. *"I don't have a space of my own in our apartment or even in my life, so I initially found it impossible to visualize a space of my own. It took me a long time to even get that far."*

For someone like Sue, the very idea of having a space that was just hers, that no one else could come into, was overwhelming at first. Even though this is an imaginary room, it may bring up other issues of your own space in your life.

Remember this room is yours and no one else can come in without your say-so.

This is your world; you are in complete control and can change everything and close the door at any time. Stay in the room as long as you feel comfortable and then leave. Just hang out with yourself; you have spent years away from this place, and now you need to make friends with it again. You may like to leave a window open so the sun can continue to stream in before you close the door behind you. Come back again and again and change whatever you like until it feels right.

Do your life breaths. Open your eyes. Spend a few moments sitting quietly, absorbing the feelings that have come up. Now write down your first impressions in your journal.

- How does the room look?
- How does it feel to be in the room?
- What do you still need to do to make it feel completely safe?
- Do you have any space that is completely yours in your real life?

Stage 4: Staying in the Room

When you are ready, open the door wide. Let the waves lap gently against the entrance, or a river run smoothly past, with a lovely view of the hills. How does the room feel today? Less cold and musty?

Open the windows wide and let the sunlight flood into the room. Think of what you still need in there to make the room yours. You might like to have some rosemary and perfumed flowers in the room in big pots, so that when you brush against them you can smell them. What about a dozen giant sunflowers in a corner of the room? Wedge a pot of scented geraniums against the door so that it stays wide open. Make a big pot of coffee so that the room is filled with the smell.

What about music? How about a baby grand in the corner so you can play your favorite jazz? Or a state-of-the-art guitar? Put your favorite CDs in the player and turn the music up loud . . . loud . . . louder still. Sing along and dance around the room . . . this is your space, do whatever seems right to make it feel comfortable and at home.

Do you like animals? Would having a pet in the room help? How many would you like? Hang your favorite paintings on the wall—Matisse, Chagall, Rembrandt. You can have the originals, this is your space! Let your imagination run wild.

After several weeks, I looked forward to coming back to the room, watering the flowers, standing in the sunlight, listening to the waves lap against the door. It felt a great relief to be there, to have reclaimed a shut-off part of my heart. I found myself spending more and more time there in my imagination—first thing in the morning, on the way to work, in my lunch hour, I'd find myself back there again.

As soon as I had ten minutes to spare, there I'd be in front of the door, admiring the paint job, peeking into the room with more and more delight at how it had changed since that first day. Or I would lie on the sofa and listen to my favorite tracks on the CD over and over, with a cup of hot fresh coffee in my hand. Or I would spend ages watering the plants and tending them, cutting flowers and putting them in vases.

The powerful thing about the room is that it is the one space in the whole world that is totally yours, totally under your control. Come back as often as you can. Make it yours and remember to keep your journal of how your feelings change as you get used to this space.

Do your life breaths. Open your eyes. Spend a few moments sitting quietly, absorbing the feelings that have come up. Now write down your first impressions in your journal.

- How does the room feel now?
- Do you find yourself thinking about it when you are not there?
- What do you still need to do to it?

Stage 5: The Forgiveness List

After some time—days, weeks, or months—the room will feel completely yours. You'll come in and water the plants, feed the cat or dog, put the music on, make yourself some tea or coffee and sit on the sofa.

Look around the room; does it feel yours and safe? When it does, it is time to imagine pinning your forgiveness lists from Chapter 2 up on one wall where you can see them. You have already taken the most difficult step—opening the door to the room and having the courage and faith to stick with it.

Now you need to spend time with the lists that you made, weeks or months ago, of the people you need to forgive and those you need to be forgiven by. Look at them again. Do they need changing? Are there people you would like to add to the easy list? Or do some people need moving from the easy list to the hard list? You will probably find that you want to add quite a few names!

Do your life breaths. Open your eyes. Spend a few moments sitting quietly, absorbing the feelings that have come up. Now write down your first impressions in your journal.

Finish with your life breaths.

When you are ready you can move on to the next stage of forgiveness. You will start by bringing one person from your easy list into the Forgiveness Room and letting them go. But the room needs to feel completely yours before you do.

6

Healing in the Forgiveness Room

You tend to feel sorrow over the circumstances instead of rage, you tend to feel sorry for the person rather than angry with him. You tend to have nothing left to remember to say about it all. You understand the suffering that drove the offence to begin with. You are not waiting for anything. You are not wanting anything. There is no lariat snare around your ankle stretching from way back there to here. You are free to go. It may not have turned out to be a happily ever after, but most certainly there is now a fresh 'Once upon a time' waiting for you from this day forward.

CLARISSA PINKOLA ESTES

$\mathcal{I}$N CHAPTER 2 you looked at your family tree of forgiveness and drew up lists of those people you need to forgive. You have also opened up the Forgiveness Room for the first time and made it completely yours. Now it's time to use that room for healing the forgiveness lists.

Begin as always with some meditation and your life breaths. Feeling nervous or scared? Many people feel that they want to bring someone from the hard list into the Forgiveness Room right away. But it is vital that you start with the easy list. Just as you got yourself used to the Forgiveness Room slowly, so it is with the healing of forgiveness itself. You need to learn how to do it properly before you can tackle the hard list.

Ground Rules

1. **You are completely safe.** No one comes in or stays without your permission. If at any time you don't feel safe or want them to leave because the process is too much for you, then they disappear immediately.
2. **You are the only person who has a say in this room.** You may ask the other person to speak as part of the healing process, but only when you are good and ready. You can't be argued with, shouted at, or contradicted here.
3. **You can refuse forgiveness.** Take as long as you like to come to healing forgiveness with someone. This applies particularly when you come to the hard list. It may take weeks or months to even allow them to stay in the room, let alone forgive them.
4. **Forgiving does not mean forgetting.** This is particularly important with the hard list. What happened to you remains true and it will always be wrong. This is your chance to let it go.

If you are doing this in a group, you may want to use one of the other group members to represent the person you need to forgive, once they come into the room and sit down. But remember that they don't get to talk.

Letting go . . . The easy list

WHEN YOU ARE ready, take yourself back to your Forgiveness Room, making sure to go through all four stages first. Do your life breaths. Now do whatever you need to feel comfortable. You may want to water the flowers, play with the dog, stroke the cat, dance around, put the music on loud, make yourself a cup of coffee.

Look at the list and pick the name of someone who has done you a very minor wrong. Choose someone you don't know personally—for example, the person who pushed in front of you in a line when you were in a rush to get home.

Now remember what happened between you, what exactly led up to the hurt. Go over the whole scene in your mind in detail. Now look out of the door and imagine a winding path coming gently up to the door. Let the person you have chosen come slowly up the path. See how the person is slightly out of breath and may be having difficulty walking. Are you ready for the person to come into the room? If you are not, and many people panic at this stage, send the person away again, until you are ready. You may need several tries before you are ready to invite anyone into the room.

Now let the person come in. Find the person a chair to sit on; you may want to give him or her a cup of coffee. Sit quietly until you are ready to talk. Then tell the person how much you have been hurt by what he or she has done or how you feel about it. Go through the story thoroughly until you are satisfied that you have told your version as clearly as you can.

Remember that the other person doesn't get to talk. The person says nothing during this time. He or she listens to you. This is a very important part of the healing process, because many people feel that their side of the story never gets heard. In the Forgiveness Room, you will always have a voice: your side of the story will always be heard loud and clear.

Seeing with better eyes

Seeing with better eyes, we can recognize that the offender is a valuable human being who struggles with the same needs, pressures, and confusions that we struggle with. We will recognize that the incident really may not have been about us in the first place.

Instead it was about the wrongdoer's misguided attempt to meet his or her own needs. As we regard offenders from this point of view (regardless of whether they repent and regardless of what they have done or suffered), we will be in a position to forgive them.

MARGARET HOLMGREN

Now you are going to change places and see it from that other person's point of view. That person still doesn't get to talk. Imagine going to stand behind his or her chair. Relive the whole scene again through that person's eyes. See how it felt to do what he or she did to you.

Feel why the person might have wanted to hurt you as he or she did. Was it accidental or just plain clumsy? Had that person had a terrible day and were you the last in line who paid for all the slights he or she had received during the day? The person may have had his or her own hurts and was trying to pass them on to you. Say out loud what you feel when you stand behind the person.

    ❧ Imagine what they were feeling just before the incident. What else had happened to make them feel like this?
    ❧ How did they first notice you and what did they think? Did they notice you at all or did you simply "get in the way?"
    ❧ What were they thinking as the incident unfolded?
    ❧ How did they feel when they saw your reaction?
    ❧ How did they feel an hour later?

Sue imagined the woman who sells her a weekly bus pass every Monday. *"She's so slow. Always holds everyone up and by the time I get to the front of the queue I'm fuming, already late for work."* Sue had no problem recounting the situation and voicing her anger at this woman that she has to deal with every week. When it came to trying to see it through her eyes, she initially found that difficult, until she came up with some questions as to why the woman might be like that every week.

"I realized that she probably commuted and had to get up really early in the morning to start work. That she might have kids she was worried about leaving to find their own way to school. That she had not been trained properly and wasn't quite sure how to do the job. That faced with a line of impatient people in a hurry she panicked and it made things even worse."

Sue still found it hard to forgive the woman. It is often difficult to forgive the first person on your list because you are learning the process. There is a voice deep inside you, warning you that if you forgive this first person, then it follows that eventually you may well forgive everyone on your list, even the hard ones. That is when you will hear a screech of brakes as you panic. But take it easy. This process has its own momentum and it has brought you this far. Trust in the journey.

So even though Sue found it hard to forgive the first person on her list, she still had a glimmer of understanding that the woman behind the ticket window had not set out to hurt her in particular. That is a crucial lesson for us to learn: the casual hurts that people we don't know inflict on us have nothing to do with us. We are simply acting as mirrors for other people's pain.

For Clare, the first person on her list was the eight-year-old boy who used to pull her hair and bully her on the bus home from school every night.

"When I stood behind Eric, the first thing that surprised me was how small he was. He'd been a giant monster in my mind all these years. We lived in the same town and I realized that he was jealous of my happy family: I was going home to a mom and dad and I was going to be talking about my day. He was going home to a violent dad and no mom; she'd died the year before. No one cared about him, he'd be lucky to get any decent meals and even luckier not to get hit when his dad came home drunk."

Many people find this exercise difficult—because it seems to allow for another version of what happened to be true. It is vital in the Forgiveness Room to know that your own version is true— particularly when we come to the hard list. It may be the only time in your life that you feel that your voice has been really heard.

Trust in the process. This exercise doesn't deny what happened to you—it allows you to see that what happened might not have been about you at all.

Once you have told your version and stood behind the other person's chair, there is now a third stage in the process. Don't stand near one chair or the other, but stand between them, so you see the story from the point of view of an outsider. Now tell the story again. See if anything new comes up when you are looking at the situation from this angle.

Clare realized that she was happy as a child and her happiness just highlighted Eric's sadness. "*He couldn't express how sad he was to have lost his mom and couldn't tell anyone how scared he was of his dad. The only thing he could do was take it out on someone who had what he didn't.*"

Now it's time to let go of this first person on your list and forgive him or her. Go back to your own chair. Now that you have seen the story from several points of view, do you feel differently about the other person? At this point it is important to be clear in your mind about exactly what forgiveness means. Remember the Forgiveness Formula:

- ๑ It means completely letting go of the hurt this person has done you.
- ๑ It means letting go of the hold this narrative has had on your life.
- ๑ It means getting rid of a piece of baggage that you will no longer have to carry around with you.
- ๑ It does not mean forgetting what has been done to you.
- ๑ It does not mean that you do not learn lessons from what happened to you.

Before you let go of the person and what he or she did to you, it's important to remember that this is the pattern of forgiveness that you will be doing over and over again with your easy and hard lists. So you must be truthfully ready to let go completely. You might like to write down what lessons you have learned from your contact with this person and what he or she did to you.

- Are they the first signs of a core issue of forgiveness (i.e. an issue that appears over and over again in your life with different people)?
- Are you scared of doing this and feel that you are not quite ready to forgive the person?
- Do you have really strong feelings coming up that have nothing to do with this person?

If you answer "yes" or even "maybe" to any of these questions—congratulations! It means that you are really engaging with the forgiveness process. This first person is a crucial step on your path of forgiveness and it is important that you get it right.

Take your time. Do some life breaths. Look the person in the eye. When you are ready, and it may take several visits to the Forgiveness Room before you feel really ready to release the bitterness, tell the person out loud that you are going to forgive him or her. That you are going to let go of the bitterness that you have held in this room of your heart all this time. You do not condone what the person has done (though having swapped places, you may understand more of the reason why) but you forgive him or her. Sit quietly with this for a moment. Feel the sensation of letting go of the bitterness in your heart. When you are ready, give the person something that represents your forgiveness—a beautiful stone, flower, or shell. And let the person go.

Watch the person go back down the path and out of your life. Now find an image of completion for yourself. It may be a beautiful shell that you place on a seashore. Let it be washed away by the tide. It may be a stick that you throw on a fire. Look at it as it catches fire and burns. Watch it go . . . it is gone. Now cross the person's name off the list that you made. Finish with your life breaths.

How does it feel to have let your first person come into the

Forgiveness Room and leave? Give yourself a few days for the feelings to sink in. You may feel relief, regret that you didn't forgive the person before, or unexpected feelings. You may find yourself having very vivid dreams about people on your hard list. You may find yourself crying more than usual or feeling particularly vulnerable and tender. Keep a diary of how your feelings change during the week; the diary will be helpful as you forgive more and more people on your list.

As you go through the easy list and begin to understand the process of forgiveness, you may find yourself zipping through the list. If you find the process suddenly gets hard, it may be because a person reminds you of someone who is on your hard list. Or it may be because you are coming smack up against the Forgiveness Paradox that we talked about on page 77. The Forgiveness Paradox is inescapable and you will have to spend much time wrestling with it.

Forgiveness is never about "them"—it's about you.
But what the person did to hurt you
may have nothing to do with you at all.

Grasping the paradox is the reason we start with the easy list— with people who did you casual or unintentional wrong.

Repeat the process with several names on your easy list until you feel completely comfortable with the process. Take your time. You may discover that you want to move some names from the minor to the major list. That is fine. If you are doing the process in a group, you may eventually be able to forgive more than one person in the two weeks between meetings. There is no need to finish the easy list before moving on to the hard list. But you must feel at ease with the process.

Letting go of those we need forgiveness from

Once you have tackled a few people from the easy list of people you need to forgive, you might want to try one person from the easy list of people you need to ask forgiveness from. The rules are the same: start with someone you don't know personally and go through the process in the same way. But you are about to learn another fundamental rule of forgiveness that most of us have conveniently forgotten—*we all need forgiveness.*

> Forgive us our trespasses as we forgive those who trespass against us.
>
> THE LORD'S PRAYER

You can't get good at forgiveness if you haven't understood that you need to be forgiven. Asking for forgiveness shows us that we get it wrong too (sometimes really badly) and gives us an insight into what it feels like to be the bad guy in the story and our need to find a way back home. We need to learn that there are all sorts of reasons for getting it wrong and that we have all behaved less well than the image we have of ourselves. That getting it wrong is part of being human. There's no way round this one, but once we understand this and accept it we open up to the possibility of forgiving everyone. If we can acknowledge that we mess up and would like to make things better, then we open the door to forgiving the other.

But it's not straightforward. This is crunch time—it's so much easier to be the victim in the forgiveness process, to be the one with "right on your side." Much harder to acknowledge that we are all human and we all make mistakes. Remember the list of reasons that people might have hurt us? Now apply that list to why *you* might have hurt the first person you picked to ask forgiveness from. Let's just go through the reasons you might have hurt them again:

- accidentally
- because the person were in the way
- because the person reminded you of someone in your past
- because you hurt so badly you had to hurt someone else
- for no good reason at all

Feeling uncomfortable yet? It's important to begin the process of asking for forgiveness now, with the easy list, if only to get us to understand that the whole forgiveness process needs to be approached with humility.

- How does it feel to be the one needing forgiveness?
- Are you embarrassed/ashamed/feeling awkward or stupid?
- Are you finding yourself trying to justify your actions (they started it)?
- Are you ready to let go of being the person at fault?

When you have gone through the different stages and feel ready, ask the person for forgiveness. Remember, the Forgiveness Room is where *your voice is heard*, so it is your choice to decide when you are ready to be forgiven—the other person will always say yes.

Now let the person go and choose a symbolic object to represent the forgiveness you have been given.

Letting go . . . The hard list

There are several issues that need to be looked at before you let the first person from the hard list into your Forgiveness Room. It may be that you have felt up till now that your holding on to what the person did to you was a witnessing of what happened. If the person abused you, you may be the only witness; he or she may never have been caught. Perhaps your hanging onto what happened feels like the only punishment the person will ever get and if you were to give that up it feels like the person would have gotten away with what he or she did to you.

Forgiveness does not mean forgetting. But not forgiving means that you are connected to the person as if by an industrial-strength rubber band. Every time you try to get away from the memory or situation, something will trigger you and you will be bounced straight back to the connection. In the Forgiveness Room, you are finally going to set yourself free. You have shared the terrible experiences with the person who committed them; now you are going to hand them back.

These things will always have happened to you and they were bad; they may even have been terrible. But by holding on to them, you are still emotionally fixed at the point that you were at when they happened. Some part of your identity is stuck in the past; in some way you have become the person "to whom these things happened." Now you are going to acknowledge them and let them go. You are going to reclaim your ability to live in the present.

I had always wanted the man who abducted me—and who would have murdered me if I had not run away—to be found and punished. Part of the preparation for forgiving him was to acknowledge that this would never happen. He might be dead, for all I knew, but he was not going to be punished for what he did to me. For years I was the only witness to what had happened. Hanging onto the pain and bitterness was my way of ensuring it was not forgotten. The only way I had of punishing him was to say, "I am here, I am alive, and I remember."

In the back of my mind I had somehow always thought that he would be brought to justice. It had seemed to me that if I kept a place of witness in my heart for what he had done, it was an acknowledgement of what had happened. I had to spend several weeks coming to terms with the fact that if I forgave him and let him go, there would be no acknowledgement from him. I would never have my day in court.

I went over and over it in my mind, started dreaming about bringing him into the Forgiveness Room (and more often than not sending him away again). Then one day I realized that the only person I was punishing by hanging onto this bitterness was myself. What an astonishing idea! All these years I had held on grimly. I didn't know if he was dead or alive and I didn't care. Now I knew that he would never be brought to court to face what he had done, that he didn't know or care whether I was hanging onto the pain, it was certainly not punishing him. But it was punishing me and I had had enough of punishing myself, of remaining connected to him.

The names on your hard list will be people who have hurt you very deeply. They may be family or friends or lovers, they may still be alive or long dead. You may not have seen them for thirty years or may still have to see them every week. The exercise is the same; we are going to bring them into the Forgiveness Room and let what they have done to you go. It will be much harder, though, than the first group of people.

Before you start, remind yourself again of the ground rules:

1. You are completely safe. No one comes in or stays without your permission.
2. You are the only person who has a say in this room.
3. You can refuse forgiveness.
4. Forgiving does not mean forgetting.

You will need to spend some time preparing for the person's visit. Keep writing in your journal. Pay attention to your dreams: write them down, because they may hold important signals for how you are doing on your forgiveness journey. You may want to try the dream exercise at the end of this chapter. Think of all the things the person did to you that require your forgiveness. Are you really ready to forgive the person and let go of the pain completely? Don't worry if you are not yet ready to forgive everyone: the Forgiveness Room is always there for you. But remember what a relief it was to let go of the smaller grievances. It will change your life if you let go of the big ones.

> He who has not forgiven an enemy has never yet tasted one
> of the most sublime enjoyments of life.
>
> LAUTER

The method of forgiving names on the hard list is much the same as the method for forgiving those on the easy list. You bring the person into the room when you are ready, tell him or her what they did to hurt you, then move to behind the person's chair and see the situation through his or her eyes. Then see it from a third point of view. Then when you are ready, let what that person did to you go.

But with the hard list, there is likely to be more than one issue. Or the bitterness and pain has been stored for so many years that the *idea* of letting it go, never mind the reality, can seem impossible. The thing to keep in mind is that there was a time in your heart and spirit *before* this bitterness and pain—and you can feel that peace again.

It is *completely your choice* when and if to forgive. You may not be ready; it may yet be too hard. If you have been abused, no one has the right to tell you that you must forgive. It is your choice and your choice alone. But remember how far you have come. The Forgiveness Room is waiting for you the moment you are ready.

But this room is yours; no one can enter without an invitation and they have to leave if and when you want them to. You are in complete control. This is essential if you are confronting people who have done you great wrong—they may have been violent, broken your heart, or abused you in some way. It probably felt as though they always had all the power. The difference is that in the Forgiveness Room, you have the control.

Linda was so worried about bringing in some members of her family who had abused her all her life that she kept sending them away before they got anywhere near the room. She had never felt safe in their presence. Then she had an idea. "*They can come in, but they have to sit here in handcuffs. Then I'll be scared, but they won't be able to hurt me.*"

At first just sitting with one of her brothers in the room was enough. Trying to make herself feel safe, she then imagined some heavy-duty bodyguards who would stand by ready for action if they were needed. And remember this is the terror that images of people in a virtual room can induce . . .

For Laura, bringing the husband who had spent much of their twenty-year relationship bullying her into the room was difficult. "*I felt I was very, very controlled, bullied, and manipulated and consequently my sense of self-esteem and value were eroded. Not in big nasty ways necessarily, although there was a fair amount of verbal abuse involved, but in lots of little things. I went on having a great amount of trouble with the idea of having him come into the room because the history of our relationship was one of my space being invaded by him and I just didn't want him in it."*

If you have been badly bullied by someone, the space you have for yourself and your own self-esteem gets smaller and smaller until you are in danger of disappearing.

"He would be standing over me saying, 'You're fucking useless because of this, that, and the other. The reason you're not a good mother is because of this and that, and it would turn into a great litany of: 'You are scum. If you would just listen to me and do what I say then I could have some respect for you.' And that just became completely intolerable. It wasn't going to get any better; I wasn't in a position to retrieve myself from this basic position of low self-esteem."

Sometimes you have such a history with the other person that getting them into the room at all feels impossible. It may be that you feel there is so much to forgive that you really don't know where to start. Or that you feel that maybe they will somehow get to take over your room and behave as badly as they did in your real relationship, particularly if you have felt powerless in the relationship. Reread the ground rules. Spend more time on your own in the room. Try bringing another person named on the easy list. If you get stuck and still find yourself just not able to bring them into the room at all, try the bonfire exercise.

Bonfire exercise

Imagine all the things that the person has done wrong to you as an enormous bonfire. Each log and stick represents one problem you have with them—big logs for big problems, sticks for the minor things, twigs for the annoyances. Build it up as high as you like; keep piling the bonfire until it represents all you need to forgive. Now pick one stick (not a log at this stage) and imagine what it represents.

For Laura it was the fact that her husband would interrupt her work and insist that she join him for lunch. "*No matter how often I got him to promise to let me get on with my work, no matter how many arguments we had about it, come lunchtime there would be that tap on the door.*"

Laura found herself spending the morning not working, dreading the lunchtime tap on the door. But remembering all the bigger things she had to forgive him for, Laura felt able to forgive him this one thing that he did, always interrupting her work so she could make him lunch.

So she took the stick that represented this, imagined a fire, and burnt it. She realized that she was able to forgive him one small hurt and that all the other hurts were just sticks and logs on the bonfire, waiting to be tackled when she was ready.

Soon she felt able to tackle a log—that her husband would often make fun of her in front of the children. "*I would go to the supermarket with the children and I would come back and go upstairs and I would hear him berating me to the children about having bought the wrong kind of cereal.*"

This was a harder log to burn, but it was still only one log, not the sum total of all the mean things he had done that she felt needed forgiveness. She decided to burn this log too and found herself giggling. He had lost his power. "*Now I can visualize him coming into the Forgiveness Room for a short period of time and feel some sense of confidence that it is my room. And if I tell him to go, he will go.*"

The "aha moment"

Sometimes the Forgiveness Room works the first time. It's like flicking a light switch on—you just get it. Chloe brought just one person into the room and something clicked. "*I just understood the process. It really helped. I realized how grudges are formed and how I stopped myself from letting go and forgiving people. Basically putting things in perspective that some things are in the past and that you can't touch the past. What has happened has happened; you can affect the future, it just depends how you behave in the present and that was important.*"

Remember that forgiving means cutting the tie that has bound you to the perpetrator all these years, that has bounced you back every time you looked like you were going to escape. When you forgive, you'll realize that you can easily slip it off and it's gone: no matter how powerful the tie is, it won't bounce you back.

**Letting go of the connection with the person
means letting go of the voice they still have loud
and clear in your head.**

This is particularly important with people who will still be in your life on a regular basis; for example, when you share custody of children.

Some people are reluctant to forgive because withholding forgiveness is the only way they feel able to maintain any sense of power. Not forgiving may feel like the only control you have ever had in the relationship. But you will find that letting go is infinitely more powerful. Other people are so caught up with remembering the difficult parts of a relationship, they can only see the person they need to forgive as a cartoon villain. If your relationship has been an ongoing one and has had good times as well as bad, you may find the following exercise helpful.

Remembering happier times

Imagine going back somewhere you were happy with the person, before he or she hurt you. For Laura, it was a swimming pool.

"I was visualizing a pool. We were there on my thirtieth birthday and it was in Italy and it was a very beautiful pool that had a natural fountain running into it. I felt happy and relaxed."

Remember being happy with the person; live out the scene fully. Now, still seeing yourself in that scene, imagine yourself as a powerful person—you may be a fire fighter, a scientist, or a doctor.

"At that moment I was thinking of myself as a professional psychologist. I even had a white coat on and glasses and looked terribly stern and professional and he was completely unable to have any negative impact on me in that state. I really felt he could say what he had to say but it would bounce off; there was nothing he could actually do to hurt me."

Now multiply out the powerful image you have chosen so that they are standing all around you and protecting you. Create as many of them as you need—dozens, hundreds, a whole football crowd of powerful "you" figures. Now choose some trivial thing that the person you need to forgive would argue with you about and you in your current state would find it very difficult to defend yourself against.

Laura was able to transfer that sense of power back into her real-life relationship. "Even very recently, I had an argument with him over the phone about letting the children stay over with some friends on a weeknight. He felt I shouldn't have done that and he called five times to try and bully me into changing my mind and having them stay with him on that night instead. I was able to imagine dozens of strong psychologist 'me's' and just say to him, 'You can't treat me like this,' and, 'This isn't going to work. This constant bullying went on in our marriage but it's not going to go on anymore.'"

To her surprise, her husband stopped trying to bully her. Now every time he tries again (after all, our familiar patterns are difficult to shake off), she imagines herself surrounded with strong images of herself and he gives up.

Imagining a different life

People from your hard list are deeply embedded in your life. So before you tackle someone from the hard list, it may be that you need to sit on your own in the Forgiveness Room with the issues that will come up if you forgive them. Try filling in the blanks.

- ❧ If I forgive him/her _____
- ❧ If I don't forgive him/her_____
- ❧ If I forgave I'd be_____
- ❧ Forgiving this means_____

Don't beat yourself up. Now more than ever you need to be gentle with yourself. Get plenty of sleep, give yourself dreaming time, make sure you do plenty of meditation. When you begin uncovering these issues you may find surprising feelings coming up of sadness or anger. Don't panic—you are preparing your heart to heal. I spent weeks in a rage of anger that felt like it might envelop me. I was grumpy with my friends and had so much energy to burn that I found myself doing fast laps of the local swimming pool—and watch out, anyone who got in my way!

It's important to stay with these feelings and not to be afraid of them. They are the sign that you are getting to the deep stuff. But it can be lonesome and isolating, so it's important to get support from your trusted friends at this point. You don't have to go into details unless you want to; just tell one or two people that you are swimming through rough water and would appreciate a little "TLC." Make sure that you choose the right people to confide in. If you are known as the strong one in your group of friends, it may scare or panic some people if you tell them that things are difficult.

If this happens, remember this is not your problem and it is not about you—though it is difficult not to see this as a rejection both of your feelings and what you are going through. Change often scares people because it reminds them of the things that they should change in their own lives. But unexpected support and allies will also appear.

Letting go . . . what do you have to lose?

Before you can think of forgiving someone from the hard list, you need to face perhaps the most difficult hurdle of all. What do you gain from hanging onto the pain? What do you have to lose if you let it go?

It sounds crazy to think that when you have been so badly hurt you would want to hang onto the pain of what happened. But we do, for all sorts of reasons. That doesn't justify the terrible things that were done to you. But when we are deeply connected to another person through a painful experience, it's like any relationship; it has both positive and negative sides. Forgiving them means letting go of the connection once and for all. These questions are probably the most difficult ones you will have to answer in your whole journey of forgiveness.

- What do I have to lose if I forgive?
- What do I gain from hanging onto the pain?
- Imagine completely letting go and forgiving . . . what does that feel like?

For me, being an innocent victim gave me an identity. I had fought back, I had survived, no one could hurt me that badly ever again. It had unintentionally become my reference point—I survived that, so I can certainly get through this. It was also a defining moment in my life: I chose to live, to fight back and survive, and fighting became my default position in any other crisis. I was wary of other people; I divided new acquaintances into those I felt I could trust and the rest. A part of me was always on duty, always, every minute of the day, on my guard against possible attack.

So what did I have to lose if I forgave? My whole way of being in the world, which had saved my life and kept me safe all these years. But it was also such a struggle being on guard twenty-four hours a day. I longed to let my guard down but didn't know how I could do that safely. The answer lay in letting go of that identity, in being open to the possibility of change, however difficult and however long it took.

Sitting in my Forgiveness Room, listening to Madonna singing "The Power of Goodbye," on the sofa with a cup of coffee in my hand, the sun streaming through the windows and the waves gently lapping at the door, I felt ready to forgive the man who had abducted me all those years ago.

I did the life breaths because I felt scared. Then I asked him to come up the hill. This was strange because I couldn't really remember what he looked like; I had only a vague memory of blondness and a suit and tie. I was terrified when he came walking up the hill; it felt like I was being transported back to the eleven-year-old who had been so deeply hurt and whose life had been changed forever by what he had done. When he got near the door I felt so scared that I had to send him away again. It took several attempts for me to feel safe enough to bring him into the room.

I sat him down on a chair opposite me and told him how I felt about what he had done. How it had changed me for life, taken away the innocence of my childhood. How what he had done had been very wrong. I knew he wasn't going to be punished but I was going to let go of the pain that had been with me all these years.

Then I found that I wasn't yet really ready to let go. I had to make him go away. I needed to sit with what he had done to me for a while longer. If I let this go, if I forgave him, what would I have left of me? It seems strange, but in a way the abduction defined me. I was the person who had survived this. In some ways it made me strong and invincible: I had chosen to live and survived. It was a grid reference on my map, a yardstick of future pain; nothing would ever be as bad again. It was so familiar, like a scar you want to pick at. Who would I be if I let it go? It felt like there would be a big gaping hole in me. It hurt too much to let it go.

No matter. Try again. Fail again. Fail better.

ANON

Weeks later I brought him back into the room. For a long time I sat and looked at him, this man who had changed my life forever. What I saw was just a man, not the monster of my childhood imagination.

Then I swapped places with him. What I found astonished me: he was just a human being in pain. Nothing else seemed to be there, just a human being completely filled with pain.

It shocked me. I understood at a very deep level that he was desperate to get rid of some of his pain, the accumulation of everything that had been done to him. And that the only way he knew how to do this was to take what had been done to him and pass it on to others. That he had most certainly been abused himself. That he was passing on the pain of that abuse in order to share some of the hurt, though in a warped and twisted way. To abuse where he had been abused, in order that someone else should know what it felt like.

I realized then that he had not gotten away with anything. Of course he should still have been punished for what he did to me and to who knows how many others. But I didn't need him to be found and punished in order to let him go. For the first time in my life, I no longer wanted to kill him or make him suffer. I felt compassion for him. What I needed to do was to stop sharing in the pain of the abuse. I sent him away again. I needed to be on my own.

I spent days revisiting the Forgiveness Room, feeling that I could never let this go. Then one day I started crying, tears that felt as if they would never end, good tears that came from deep inside. I knew I was ready. I took another five life breaths and brought him back up the hill.

Then I sat back in my chair and said that I was going to let go of what he had done to me. It felt very scary. I took several more life breaths and told him that what he had done was very wrong, but that I was now going to let it go. That all these years I had accepted the burden of sharing his pain but that was now over. I pictured myself returning a huge bundle of pain, giving it back to him. I showed him outside to where there was a huge fire and got him to burn it on his own. Then he left, walking back down the hill.

I let the sea wash soothingly against the door and sat and cried for a long time. Then when I was ready I crossed his name off the list and I took the most beautiful shell I had and gently put it on the shore and let it be washed away.

Now several years later, reading the account of forgiving my abductor still sends a shiver down my spine. It took so many years to get there, but when I did the forgiveness was absolute and final. And my life changed. What I discovered was that forgiving him allowed what had happened to be acknowledged in other ways. We were no longer bound together by the secret. I could begin to tell my story to more of my tried and trusted friends. It was out in the open and it had finally lost its power. I also found I didn't need to stand guard all the time. At first this was scary, because it felt as though anyone could attack me and I would not be protected. But when someone did go for me at work, I discovered to my surprise that I was still perfectly capable of defending myself. I just didn't need to be on full alert all the time anymore.

Taking your core issues into the Forgiveness Room

In Chapter 3 we looked at how we can begin to forgive the past and let it go. And how that brings up the core issues of forgiveness that we all have, issues that come up again and again with different people, until we realize that they represent a key event from our forgiveness past that needs to be resolved. The person who planted your core issue in your heart will appear somewhere on your hard list of forgiveness.

Once you have identified what your core issue is and where it came from in your past, you will need to take it into the Forgiveness Room.

Bring the person who caused this to become your core issue into the room and take him or her through the forgiveness process.

When you have forgiven that person and let him or her go, it is time to forgive the core issue itself and let it go. Because it has taken on a life of its own in your narrative and become separated from the person who first caused it to become a problem, you need to forgive it too.

Try to find an image that symbolizes your core issue. It might be a poster with the lettering written out in capital letters. Or an object that takes you straight back to the core issue. Some people find a symbol helpful. I used a picture of an ear for my "being listened to" core issue and a Girl Guide badge for the reliability symbol.

Now put the image on the chair opposite you and take it through the same forgiveness process. You might like to thank the core issue for the positive things it has given you (for example, mine have made me utterly reliable and a good listener). Then take it through the ways it has been less helpful. When you are ready to let it go, tell it so and that you are going to forgive it. Then find a creative way of destroying the symbol.

Forgiveness in the present

But what if the person you need to forgive is still present in your life, perhaps a partner or a parent? How is it possible to forgive and get whatever behavior is calling for forgiveness to stop? The same rules apply in the Forgiveness Room, but with a slight twist.

First you have to be very clear that from this day forward, whatever abusive behavior has happened in the past must stop. The person will not abuse you, in whatever way, from now on. You will be in control. Of course the person may well try the old ways—you must remember that it is you who has changed, not them—but the fact that you *have* changed alters the whole situation. You will no longer be accepting the person's behavior and will take steps to make sure that it is not reproduced. This may involve putting distance between you and the other person. You may or may not choose to tell the person of your decision, and you may want to tell someone else about the abuse. But to forgive the person, you must first protect yourself.

When a person is still present in your life, there are two separate issues to face. Forgiveness of past behavior and what to do about the future: how to stop the person from doing what hurts you. It is even more important when you are doing this exercise with someone who is still present in your life that you should take things slowly. Don't rush the process in the Forgiveness Room, or it won't work. Don't be afraid to take weeks, even months, with each stage.

Bring the person into your Forgiveness Room and do the same exercises. Take yourself through all the same stages as the others on your list. If you feel like stopping and running away, go back a stage and take the life breaths.

When you let the person go, you need to work out a way of showing the person in the real world that things are now different. It is completely up to you how you handle things. There is no need to tell the person you have forgiven him or her, though you may eventually find it helpful. Notice how differently you feel when you are with the person: you have let go of past pain, but you still need to deal with the present and the future.

The person may sense you want to change the relationship and feel very uncomfortable; it may even accentuate the abusive behavior. You have to be ready and firm in your resolve to protect yourself.

It may be that you have to spend less time with the person. It may be that you will one day have the courage to have the same conversation with him or her in real life—though of course you will be less in control, as the person will be able to react.

You may need to tell someone else if you are being abused in some way; you certainly need to make it clear to the real person that things are different now. Practice on the imaginary person in your room: what do you think his or her reaction will be? Practice what your reaction will be. At this point, if you are doing this in a group it may be helpful to have input from the others. Get one of them to be the person you are struggling with so that you can practice your reactions.

The most important thing is to ensure your safety. You have the right to be safe from physical and mental abuse. But the situation may be very complicated, so take your time. You will be astonished that when you change, the world changes with you. You are no longer the victim; you now have a say in the world.

After Forgiveness

When you have crossed people off your list in the Forgiveness Room, you may feel like contacting the real person. It is a good idea not to do this right away. You may not need to tell the person anything, because the way you behave now will be different and that will change the dynamic of your relationship anyway.

Just as you took things slowly in the Forgiveness Room, you need to do the same in your real life. Providing you are safe from immediate danger, take your time. Set up good support structures, get help from your friends and family, your pastor, your doctor, or other agencies. The more trusted people are aware of the situation, the greater support you will have to make the changes to your life that you need.

It may be that the person you need to forgive has an indirect effect on your life; maybe the person has a problem with drugs, gambling, alcohol, or some other addiction. Maybe the person is terrible with money and this has a catastrophic effect on your life. Perhaps the person is so taken up with his or her own pain that the person just wishes you to have some of it.

When you bring the person into the Forgiveness Room, take his or her chair for a while and see the world through that person's eyes. It will surprise you. This is not in any way to excuse or condone that person's behavior, but it will help you understand him or her better, which in turn will allow you to cope better with the change.

The important thing to remember is that once you change, nothing will ever be the same again.

An exercise for those finding it difficult to engage with the process of forgiveness

The unblocking exercise

Begin as always with some meditation to leave the outside world behind and get yourself to a peaceful place. Now do some life breaths.

This is an adaptation of an exercise that was first developed by Saint Ignatius, who started the Jesuit movement. He broke his leg, but it wasn't set very well and left a lump that showed through his tights. Being vain, he decided to have the leg re-broken (without the benefit of anesthetic!) and during a long convalescence he developed a series of spiritual exercises. This is one of them.

Read the following parable several times. If you don't come from a Christian tradition, you may find it more helpful to substitute your own holy figure for Jesus—Buddha, the Goddess, an inspiring character from your favorite book—the important thing is that it should be a being of pure love.

> Now there is in Jerusalem by the Sheep Gate a pool, in Hebrew called Bethzatha, which has five porticoes. In these lay a multitude of invalids, blind, lame, paralyzed. The ancient authorities tell us that they were waiting for the water to move; for an angel of the Lord went down at certain seasons into the pool and troubled the water. Whoever stepped in first after the troubling of the water was healed of whatever disease he had.
>
> One man was there who had been ill for thirty-eight years. When Jesus saw him and knew that he had been lying there a long time, he said to him, "Do you want to be healed?" The sick man answered him, "Sir, I have no man to put me into the pool when the water is troubled and while I am going, another steps down before me." Jesus said to him, "Rise, take up your pallet and walk." And at once the man was healed and he took up his pallet and walked.[1]

Now you are going to imagine yourself within the parable. You are going to be there and imagine what happens. Look around you—what does the pool look like? Describe the scene to yourself.

Now go over to the paralytic and speak to him. The holy figure comes over and talks to the paralytic—what does he look like? How does he seem, what is he wearing? Now you have a chance to talk to the holy figure. He turns to you and asks you the same question, "Do you want to be healed?" Over to you . . .

When I first did this exercise I was astonished. First, standing among all the people with terrible physical things wrong with them and standing by the paralytic, I realized that I felt it would never be my turn. That my wounds were not visible and it seemed that there was a long line of people in front of me who would get there first.

Then when Jesus asked me if I wanted to be healed, I realized that I couldn't say yes. Could I let go? Could I be different? I found that I couldn't ask to be healed, I wasn't yet willing.

Over the months I used this exercise as a way of seeing how I had moved on, taking myself through the whole process each time. I got to walk with Jesus in the olive groves near the pool and we talked. Eventually it changed me and allowed me to really engage with the process of forgiveness.

After a while I realized I had operated on the flight/fight mode all my life. What was different now was that I was no longer running, but really present. That left me with the possibility of fight. I spent several weeks furiously angry, accessing rage that seemed to come from deep within, and I didn't see how I could give up my anger. If I did, it felt like I would be left with nothing. I did the parable imagery again and Jesus asked me if I wanted to be healed of the anger. I said maybe we could let go of half of it as a test! He smiled so gently and I asked what I would be without the anger to defend me. "You would be free," He said—and that word resonated through me.

Notes

[1] *Holy Bible: New International Version*: John 5.2–10

7

Overcoming
Some Obstacles
to Forgiveness

Hope for a great sea-change
On the far side of revenge.
Believe that a further shore
Is reachable from here.
Believe in miracles
And cures and
Healing wells.

SEAMUS HEANEY

A sense of justice

WITHOUT A SENSE of justice, forgiveness can seem impossible. But often the person you need to forgive cannot be punished or even confronted. So the offence is open-ended, without resolution. That is often a place where we get stuck. So how do you achieve a sense of justice to enable you to engage with the process of forgiveness? And what happens if you don't manage to arrive at some sense of justice?

Justice appeals to our deepest sense of what is fair. We all have a sense of natural justice, of right and wrong. It is deeply offensive to that basic emotion to feel that there is no comeback against someone who has done something wrong. There is a sense of a double wrong, that someone has not just committed an offence but effectively gotten away with it. Ask yourself how you feel about even these trivial examples:

- someone not paying his or her fare on the bus
- someone pushing in front of you in a line when you have been waiting for ages
- a sports figure found to be taking performance-enhancing drugs.

A sense of justice is crucial to our feeling that the world is a fair place. Otherwise our moral universe makes no sense. We all have a code that we live by, a set of rules that governs how we behave in the world and how we expect others to behave. When that code is broken, it can leave us with a strong sense of injustice.

Holding on to the sense of injustice

George is a quiet man, a painter in his sixties. Recently he said to me that only two people in his life had really done him a great wrong—and he could forgive neither. One of them had subsequently died but he still didn't forgive him. What was startling was the anger in his voice when he talked about them and the hurt; they were still bonded by whatever had happened.

If you don't feel able to reach a sense of justice, you may be haunted by the desire for revenge. You may find yourself playing out the scenario again and again in your head, in ways in which you get to react differently. You may have violent dreams or fantasies about the person, in which you hurt or even kill them. This does not make you a terrible person; they are an expression of your frustration, the depth of your hurt and anger. As we can see across the world, revenge brings no sense of satisfaction; it merely continues the cycle of pain.

> If we practice an eye for an eye and a tooth for a tooth, soon the whole world will be blind and toothless.
>
> MAHATMA GANDHI

Though it is completely understandable—we want the offender to feel a part of the pain that he or she has imposed on us—it does not seem to work. If it did, warring communities across the world would have found peace. But they clearly haven't. And revenge can leave even the temporary satisfaction with a bitter taste.

Stephanie discovered that her husband of thirty years had been having an affair with her best friend. She threw them both out of her life but was eaten up with anger and the desire for revenge. "*So one night I got out the kitchen knife and walked over to their apartment. I found her car and slashed all four tires. The satisfaction it gave me when I heard the sssshhhh sound of the air coming out was amazing. I knew they would know it was me without being able to prove it.*"

The problem is that Stephanie is telling me this story five years later and she still remembers and savors every detail. The couple is still together and she has lost her husband and best friend. She has become completely obsessed not with the affair, but with the consequences, demanding that any common acquaintances must take sides—her side. It is also her only topic of conversation. Far from giving her any peace, slashing the tires has fueled her hunger for revenge and satisfaction.

Longing for the past to be different

What Stephanie really wants is for everything to be as it was before; it's as though her brain is unable to compute the changed situation, so she is stuck with what has been done to her. She knows that her friends are sympathetic but tired of hearing about it. *"I can see in their eyes that they are bored with the whole thing. But what else can I do? To give up would be like saying that what they did was all right, but it wasn't. I lost my husband and best friend. If I shrug my shoulders and say it doesn't matter, they'll have got away with it. I couldn't bear it."*

Stephanie has fallen into the classic trap of not being able to let go of what has happened because she feels that no one has been punished. It seems to her that they have gotten away with it. By grimly hanging on to the story, telling it at every opportunity to whoever will listen, she believes that she is punishing them. More than that, that she is the only punishment that they will get. So it becomes imperative not to give up, not to change, not to move on. But the sad thing is that the only person she is punishing is herself.

Bringing change into the world

Sometimes people react to horrific and unjust events in their lives by trying to make sure that the same thing doesn't happen to anyone else. Campaigning can be a positive way to achieve a sense of justice, both for the person lost and for the more general good. So a mother whose child has been killed by a drunk driver will set up a campaign to stop drinking and driving; families whose members have been murdered will themselves campaign against the death penalty. The group "Murder Victims' Families for Reconciliation," based in Cambridge, Massachusetts, puts it clearly: *"Reconciliation* means accepting you cannot undo the murder but you can decide how you want to live afterward."

For Denise Green, whose son William was one of the children involved in the Alder Hey scandal, and whose story we talked about on pages 70–72, a sense of justice has been important in coming to terms with their tragedy. The hospital apologized, but that was not enough. *"'Sorry' was the first step. People needed to own up and be honest about what had happened. But it had to be put right. We wanted it put right; 'sorry' was not enough—we needed to put action behind words."* Denise began to campaign for a change in the law governing the way doctors need to ask permission from parents to remove and retain the organs of dead patients.

She is clear about what justice means for her family and for William, and although she has forgiven the people who did this to her son, for her sense of justice to be satisfied, she needs some restitution. *"Some people think that if you forgive, it means you don't want justice. That isn't true. Justice for me will come when they establish a new law of consent with penalties attached. We can't undo what has been done, but we can stop it from being done again."*

Can we do things differently?

Our gut instinct tells us that to forgive we need a sense of justice. Traditionally justice has meant punishment—and we are encouraged to believe that when someone has done us wrong, the person needs to be punished before we can forgive him or her. That there is a debt to be paid. Forgiveness seems contingent on having our day in court, having our say. But what if we could achieve a sense of justice by other means?

When Nelson Mandela came to power, he recognized the need for forgiveness and led by example, inviting one of his prison guards to his inauguration ceremony. Here was a man who had spent much of his life in prison, choosing the route of forgiveness. But how could a country that had suffered so much under apartheid move forward into reconciliation? Revenge seemed a much more likely route, particularly as the perpetrators were unlikely ever to come to justice, as much evidence had been lost. It was as though the whole country needed its "day in court."

We would normally expect people who had committed the terrible acts of violence catalogued under the apartheid regime to be brought to court and punished. That is how our system of justice has been set up—punishment has become synonymous with justice.

The Truth and Reconciliation Commission in South Africa showed us one possible and different route—restorative justice. In the more traditional approach to justice, the offender is seen as having committed an offence against the state. Victims generally have very limited opportunity to say how they have been affected by the crime and the justice system keeps victims and offender apart while others speak for them. Restorative justice sees the harm done by crime as an offence against a person or organization. It allows victims the opportunity to participate, by bringing victims and offenders together, with an impartial mediator to consider from all points of view what has happened and find out what can be attempted to help put it right.

"One of the people was a woman from Soweto, Thandi, who was tortured while in detention. She was raped repeatedly. She said she survived by taking her soul and spirit out of her body and putting them in a corner of the cell in which she was being held. She could then, disembodied in this manner, look on as they did all those awful things to her body intended to make her hate herself as they had told her would happen. She could imagine then that it was not she herself but this stranger suffering the ignominy heaped on her. She then uttered words filled with deep pathos. She said with

tears in her eyes that she had not yet gone back to that room to fetch her soul and that it was still sitting in the corner where she had left it."[1]

Justice is not the same as punishment.

People who had been involved in crimes in South Africa were invited to come forward and apply for amnesty, under certain conditions. Desmond Tutu, who headed the Truth and Reconciliation Commission, believes that it proved to be a better way of getting at the truth than court cases. *"Amnesty applicants had to demonstrate that they had made a full disclosure to qualify for amnesty, so the normal legal process was reversed as applicants sought to discharge the onus on them to reveal all."*[2]

Full disclosure was the key to the process. Applicants were not required to express contrition or remorse but had to make full disclosure. In return for full disclosure of the crime, individuals were granted amnesty—the so-called "third way."

The Truth and Reconciliation Commission was never going to be able to solve all the crimes of the apartheid years in South Africa. Seven thousand people came forward to ask for amnesty. Twenty thousand people came forward to give evidence of gross violation of their human rights; about one in ten testified publicly. Although the cases are not matched one to one, it is clear that many victims had no one come forward to admit to the crimes perpetrated against them.

Some people, including commentators in South Africa, feel that the process itself was flawed. They feel that those asking for amnesty, often the perpetrators of terrible crimes, effectively "got away with it" simply by coming forward and admitting what they had done. This raises the fundamental question of how we define justice. How is justice served in this way? Was amnesty in return for complete disclosure of the crime effectively protecting the perpetrators? Was it making victims of the crime suffer needlessly?

Perhaps it is more helpful to ask how justice would have been served otherwise. The perpetrators of crimes who appeared before the Commission were never going to be brought to trial—their victims were often dead and there was very little evidence, other than the personal testimony of the survivors. Those victims who had no one come forward to testify still got to tell their stories. When the alternative was no justice at all, the Truth and Reconciliation Commission was at least trying to bring forgiveness into the equation.

So what effect did it have on the victims to be able to face their perpetrators and have their story validated in public? Here is what one young man, Lucas Sikwepere, said after he had described how a notorious Cape Town police officer had shot him in the face, blinding him: *"I feel what . . . has brought my sight back, my eyesight back, is to come here and tell the story. I feel what has been making me sick all the time is the fact that I couldn't tell my story. But now . . . it feels like I've got my sight back by coming here and telling you the story."* [3]

Desmond Tutu himself has said that he found some of the accounts unbearable and that they put a great strain on all the Commission members, but they all felt that the future of their country depended on the truth being heard and witnessed. Inadequate though the process might be, there could be no reconciliation without the truth being heard.

"Without being melodramatic, it is not too much to claim that it is a matter of life and death. On its success does hinge the continued existence of our nations, of all of us as a people and as separate individuals. It is ultimately in our own best interest that we become forgiving, repentant, reconciling, and reconciled people, because without forgiveness, without reconciliation we have no future." [4]

Coming to a sense of justice in your own life

One of the most difficult things we have to learn in life is that we don't always get justice, that bad things go unrecognized and unpunished. It offends our sense of what it means to be human. The person who did you serious harm may never face the real justice that you would like. What are you going to do about it? You have a choice: to hang on to your very real sense of grievance or find a way to let it go. So is hanging on giving you the peace you long for? Let's ask that question again.

Is it working for you?

For many of us, hanging on to our sense of grievance can be a way of hanging on to the identity of victim. It is not what happened to you, but what you do with that information. It may well be that the person who wronged you will not be punished or brought to any sort of satisfactory justice in your eyes. So how are you going to cope with that? You have two courses of action ahead—hang on to your anger and bitterness or try to come to a sense of justice yourself. You may still need to hang on to your sense of injustice for a while longer. But do it consciously, examine it, spend some time with it, and see if it really works for you.

Sometimes it seems that there is no way out. We are tied together with that familiar industrial-strength rubber band. It's a vicious circle that we are spinning round in with the offender. No possibility of punishment means no sense of justice, which in turn means no potential for letting go and cutting the connection. Often we feel that our holding on is the only punishment, so how can we let go?

Letting go of the hope of the past being different

It is often difficult to let go of the terrible things that may have happened to us because they become defining moments in our lives. So we will always be people to whom this terrible event happened. But achieving a sense of justice means that we are no longer stuck there; we acknowledge what happened and we get to let it go. If that sense of justice is missing we can remain connected to the people who have hurt us badly in our lives despite ourselves.

The only person who can change is you yourself.

For me, recognizing that the man who abducted me would never be punished was a long and painful journey. I felt trapped—if what he did to me was never recognized, then he would never be punished; he'd have gotten away with it.

The only way I could see of punishing him was to hang on vividly to the memory of what he had done, to say, "I remember, I am still here and alive and I remember what you did," in the unconscious hope that somehow there would be a day in court. I couldn't let go.

Anytime I heard on the news of a child being kidnapped, my heart would go cold. I'd be right back there, experiencing the terror and fear of being murdered. Not just remembering but experiencing the terror—cold and sweaty, heart pounding, unable to breathe. And when the parents would appear tearfully on television appealing for their child's safe return, I would see my parents there, imagining how they would have felt. Seeing the inevitable happy portrait of the child splashed across the papers the next day would be almost unbearable. I would imagine what photograph of me my parents would have used. If, unhappily, a body was found and the distraught parents were interviewed, I would see myself there, my parents and brother and sister crying for me.

It took many years for me to realize that I was not punishing him, I was punishing myself. It then took many visits to the Forgiveness Room to let it go.

My sense of justice eventually came from really understanding that I didn't need to hold onto the memory in order to punish him. That by holding on so strongly, the only person being punished was me. I no longer feared being abducted as an adult, but it seemed that I would be forever connected to the man. I could not have imagined a time when I could have let that memory go, yet when I forgave him it was as though I had taken a pair of scissors and cut the elastic that tied us together. That doesn't mean that I have forgotten. Or that when I see a couple of tearful parents on television appealing for the safe return of their daughter, I don't feel for them. But my heart no longer pounds—the image has lost its power over me.

Luke, who was repeatedly sexually abused as a child by one of his teachers, is very clear about the importance of justice—and how it is a separate issue from forgiveness. He eventually went to the police twenty years later and the man was found to have abused other boys too; the teacher was then arrested and charged with sexual offences. He eventually pleaded guilty and was put on the sex offenders register.

"Justice is a very separate issue from forgiveness. At some level you have to feel a sense of justice before you can come to forgiveness. And that means justice for everyone involved. Justice is important; in forgiving in the first place I sought justice for myself.

First and foremost within myself. I then sought justice for the child within myself. I then sought justice for myself living in society, that I would be free from this man."

Luke has forgiven the man who abused him but nevertheless believes in the importance of that man being brought to trial. So his forgiveness is inextricably linked to a sense of justice, which he believes has a ripple effect through society.

"In taking the case to trial, I'm seeking a wider justice not only for a topic such as pedophilia, but also for the people who live in the area where this man lives, and also a justice for him. Somewhere down the line there's a justice for this man's life, that he can receive help or look into the dark chasms of his life and maybe a little bit of light can be shone."

Actions have consequences

Forgiveness is a journey, not an automatic reflex. However much we practice, people will still come along in our lives who do us a wrong that profoundly affects our sense of justice. Sometimes when people act in this way, we need to learn from the situation. It may be that the relationship is changed for ever. That does not mean we should not work hard at forgiving them. It does mean we should protect ourselves so that it does not happen again. Otherwise you can be sure it will happen again until you learn the lesson. They may shed light on an area of forgiveness in your life that you need to examine. Has a similar situation happened to you before? If you react strongly, what does it remind you of?

Simon was trying to buy an apartment from a friend he had known for more than twenty years. She is the widow of one of his closest friends who died ten years ago and he had always kept an eye on her and her children as they were growing up.

"She pulled out of the deal at the last minute and took the apartment off the market.

I later discovered that she had put it on the market again for one hundred thousand dollars more. I really felt disgusted; it was like the violation of codes of honor between friends."

When a sense of injustice happens, the first and normal reaction is anger. With friends there may be a sense of coming to the end of the road in the relationship, that they have gone too far to be able to return to a position of trust. If we have felt close to someone, particularly if we have seen the person through hard times, the betrayal can feel unbearable, but we need to remember that *forgiveness is a journey;* you need to take it at your own speed. It may take months or years to even feel you can start on the journey. A year later, Simon has not yet managed to take that first step. And at the moment he is prepared to lose all the wonderful things that the friendship brought him.

"Once I have decided to send someone into the outer darkness, there is no way back. Maybe if I were more mature, I would make peace but then I think, Damn you, why should I? A nobler, more mature person might make peace."

Once the trust has been lost, making peace can seem like leaving yourself open to be taken advantage of again. Clare lost a friend when he was supposed to let her into a mutual friend's house to stay. *"It was New Years' Day and freezing cold. There was no way I could get in touch with him. I stood on that freezing doorstep for an hour, expecting him to come around the corner any minute with an excuse and a smile. But he never did. In the end I went to the local bar and left a message on the answering machine and after about two hours, someone else happened to come home and let me in. He never did turn up."*

When Clare did get hold of Bob, he was not even apologetic. *"It was unbelievable. I was so angry, and all he could say was, "Well you got in eventually, what's all the fuss about?" When he realized how hurt and angry I was he did try to apologize, but it was too late; the trust had been broken and we are no longer friends. People did try to bring us back together, but every time I looked him in the* eye, I'd remember that he was happy to leave me on that freezing doorstep for hours. And I knew he would do it again without the slightest hesitation, because he didn't really see what all the fuss was about."

If it is not resolved, we often find we break off the relationship. That may be the right thing to do at the time to protect ourselves. Of course that still leaves the problem of broken trust and forgiveness. We may be able to forgive the action and still not feel able to continue the relationship. If we happen to meet up with the person again, it can be surprising to discover how strong the feelings still are. Clare bumped into Bob at a wedding. "It was awkward; he tried to be all friendly and it was embarrassing. Later on when we had all had a bit to drink, he even pretended that he couldn't remember what it was that we had fallen out about. That made me really angry! I told him the story again and he was obviously surprised that I could remember it in such detail. I was surprised at how angry I still was about it all—the feelings of anger and betrayal were right there again as soon as the subject came up. He was very much of the 'water under the bridge' school, but this was my bridge and it felt like he was just going to get away with it if I didn't say, 'No, you did this and because of it we are no longer friends.' For me trust is central to any relationship and how could I trust him again?"

Letting go of the injustice of death

How do you square those difficult feelings of injustice when someone you love has died? How do you forgive them for leaving you and dying?

There are five recognized stages to any loss and that includes the death of a loved one:

- denial
- anger

- bargaining
- depression
- acceptance

In their book *Life Lessons: Two Experts on Death and Dying Teach Us About the Mysteries of Life and Living*, Elisabeth Kübler-Ross and David Kessler explain how loss touches us all differently.

"Not everyone goes through these five stages with every loss, the responses don't always occur in the same order, and you may visit stages more than once . . . Whatever you are feeling when you lose someone or something is exactly what you are supposed to be feeling. It is never our place to tell someone, 'You have been in denial too long, it is now time for anger,' or anything like that, for we don't know what someone else's healing should look like."

The feeling of injustice arises naturally as part of the grieving process. Someone has been taken away from us before we were ready, so it is natural that there is a sense of unfinished business. Because we can't bring the person back, the sense of unfinished business and all the other difficult feelings become attached to the person who has died. Remember that this is part of the grieving process and give yourself the time you need to heal—forgiveness will come.

Justice in the family

Children naturally have a strong sense of justice. They will often protest that an adult decision "is not fair." We can all remember situations as children when we were unfairly blamed for something by a parent or child and the sense of outrage we felt. This sense of natural justice is a good starting place to teach children that they can deal with arguments in a way that leaves both sides feeling satisfied, and the most important key to that is for both of them to be heard. The idea of "things being put right" is central to justice and the possibility of forgiveness. This is something that we need to learn early as children. A sense of justice is crucial to the settling of the daily arguments within a family.

In family situations it is important to feel a sense of justice when things go wrong. Parents don't always handle the situation in the best way possible; they may themselves have unresolved issues with justice and forgiveness and it may be too painful for them to deal with.

Chloe remembers many such occasions with her sister. *"When I was in my early twenties, my sister didn't want to give me back some clothes that I had lent to her. I wanted them back and she pretended I had given them to her and she wouldn't give them back. So I asked my mom to tell my sister to give them back and she refused and because of that I stopped talking to my mom for three months. I would just not say a word to her. She tried to talk to me but I just wouldn't speak to her at all. In the end we had a mouse in the house and we had to get together to solve the situation; otherwise we probably would still not be talking. I was so wrapped up in anger, it was hard practically but I was so angry with the whole situation."*

In leaving the children to fend for themselves, the mother had not given the tools to resolve confrontation positively.

The other day on the train, two sisters, aged about eight and six, were quarrelling in the way siblings do. The older sister kept poking and teasing and laughing at the younger sister until she got a reaction. Or she would accidentally bump her or pinch her. The younger sister would then bump her or pinch her back and soon one or both of them were in tears, or hurt or sulking, and the parents would intervene. This same scenario went on for half an hour until they got off the subway. What was astonishing was the way that the parents waited until the quarrelling had escalated and they were both in tears or yelling at each other. Occasionally the mother would say, "Girls!" in a voice that seemed to hope it would all stop magically on its own.

The girls had learned some clear lessons from their parents. That they would only intervene when things got out of hand and then only to quiet it all down. And more importantly, that there was no justice. It didn't matter who had started it, who had continued it, or who was now finishing it, they were told to be quiet and settle down. So the real problems between the sisters, what was making them pick on each other continually, were never addressed. They were learning very early in life that where their parents were concerned, there was no justice, only equal blame.

If the arguments and frustrations of family life are not resolved as they go along, then the same issues will resurface again and again until they are resolved.

Parents will say the children are always arguing about the same thing. What the children are really doing is trying to resolve the problem by bringing it up again and again. But because they don't have the emotional tools to resolve the issue, all they can do is play out the scene of battle repeatedly until the adult world notices. Then parents stop the fight, or punish both sides without getting to the bottom of the issue—what are the children trying to resolve here?—and children learn the important and unfortunate lesson that conflict doesn't get resolved, you just have to fight harder to get your voice heard. Then you get into the inevitable "she started it, no he did," "did, didn't" scenario, which resolves nothing and leaves both sides unhappy.

Cool off first

The heat of the moment is never a good time to sort arguments out. Justice is best served in a cool and calm atmosphere, which is why it is probably a good idea to have a cooling-off period so that both sides can think about what has happened. Even ten minutes will allow both sides to calm down—getting both sides to go into separate rooms or one into the yard, and actively saying, "Let's all calm down and come back in ten minutes." It will give you a chance to calm down too. Then when you come back to the table, the important thing is to let everyone be heard.

Cindy, a mother of four, found that making sure that everyone was heard was difficult. *"We developed a system where the person speaking was not to be interrupted. They were given a beautiful stone that we found on the beach once and while they held the stone, they had the floor. The kids loved the idea of being able to speak without being interrupted themselves but it was hard at first to get them not to interrupt others!"*

Being heard . . . using the "other chair"

Once everyone has told their side of the story, it helps if you can step back yourself (which is why the ten-minute time out is so helpful to you too) and ask them what they think is fair. Maybe one of them needs to say sorry; more than likely all parties in the argument need to apologize. The most important lesson children then learn is that their voice is respected, that they are listened to, and that conflict can be resolved without violence or sulking but by hearing what the other person has to say.

You might like to introduce the "other chair" technique. Get each child to imagine what it is like to have been the other child in that situation. You will find that children are naturally fair-minded and will admit when they have been in the wrong if they can do so in an atmosphere that is free from anger and blame.

It might even be helpful to get children to play with the idea of the Forgiveness Room in different ways. You could start off with the idea of a family Forgiveness Room that you all decorate and imagine together. Then the person holding the stone holds the power in the room and gets to bring the other person in and tell that person how he or she felt. They see it from their chair and then you allow the other child to do the same. See if they are ready to forgive. You will be surprised how quickly children will forgive if they feel that their voice is heard and that their natural sense of justice is understood.

Without this sense of justice, there can be no forgiveness. It is crucial that children learn how to speak the language of forgiveness as early as possible, to understand how good it feels both to forgive and be forgiven, effectively to wipe the slate clean. If you think it's not important, remember how many siblings maintain frosty relationships or no longer really have any contact because of unresolved quarrels of childhood.

Parents must encourage a spirit of forgiveness by being ready to ask their children for forgiveness when they get it wrong too. A healthy family will be able to admit that we all get it wrong sometimes, all lose our tempers, all do things we later regret. What is important is not the act itself, but being able to learn from our mistakes. Someone who always has to be in the right will find it hard to make relationships later on in life.

Coming to a sense of justice is crucial if we are really to leave the past behind and open the door to forgiveness. Understanding that we need to recognize and give full importance to what has happened to us before letting it go is central to the process. If not we will be doing ourselves a final injustice—getting caught up in the narrative of our past rather than learning to let it go.

Forgiveness in the wider world

Letting go of the past hurts. But we have seen how to bring forgiveness into our lives. Now it is time to take that forgiveness into the wider world. This time, however, we are not talking about forgiving individuals but about forgiving groups or organizations that have done you wrong. So how do you apply the Forgiveness Formula to your place of work or bank, your garage or church?

What we need to understand is that the conflicts and battles in the world are only the reflection of our own daily battles and conflicts magnified. It is an uncomfortable thought that world peace begins with us, today, in the here and now, but I believe that the forgiveness we bring to our own lives directly affects conflicts and wars across the world. If we can forgive and ask for forgiveness in the wider circles of our own lives, then any conflict can be resolved. If you still hold a grudge against your school, your bank, your church, your mechanic, then you are directly contributing to conflict in the world. If you can't forgive another religious or ethnic group, then you are directly contributing to conflict in the world. It is that simple.

In the last few years many national and symbolic figures have asked for forgiveness for wrongs committed in the name of the organization or state that they headed. From President Clinton to the Pope, from leading figures in the conflict in Northern Ireland to members of religious communities in Africa, there is a recognition that the first step to forgiveness in the wider world is learning to say sorry. Even if it is sorry for an action that took place years, or even hundreds of years in the past, and for which the present holders of the post can have no individual responsibility. This cuts right against the grain of the traditional political mantra "never explain, never apologize" and shows that there is growing recognition that forgiveness is the key to peace.

If national and religious leaders can ask for forgiveness, how can we as individuals forgive in the wider world? How do you forgive a nation, a religion, school, or bank that has done you wrong? How do you come to terms with forgiving a hospital or even the organization where you work?

Let's look at the Forgiveness Formula again and see how we can apply it to groups or organizations that have done us wrong.

- ❧ It means completely letting go of the hurt this person has done you.
- ❧ It means letting go of the hold this narrative has had on your life.
- ❧ It means getting rid of a piece of baggage that you will no longer have to carry around with you.
- ❧ It does not mean forgetting what has been done to you.
- ❧ It does not mean that you do not learn lessons from what happened to you.

As we have already seen in the section on justice, forgiveness needs the recognition that wrong has been done. Yet in an organization it is often difficult to find any single individual to admit the organization they worked for was wrong. This is increasingly the case when there is any danger of legal action.

Letting go of the hold this narrative has on your life

Many people spend their lives going over the battles of the past with their bank or some other group. They may well have been right in the original argument, but it comes to dominate their lives. They focus all their attention on writing letters to the papers or their congressperson until the original complaint is forgotten. The battle becomes a focus for all the other disappointments in their lives.

Of course we should protest against injustice in our lives and in the wider world. Changes in the world have often only come about because one brave person was willing to stand up and say, "This is not right." But the key is knowing which battles to fight. A point of principle can sometimes get lost in the desire to win and be vindicated, to be told for once that you were right.

Ask yourself these questions:

- Am I continuing this for the sake of it—for the need to be right?
- Is this battle having a direct effect on my nearest and dearest?
- Is this a battle I can win?
- In ten years' time will it matter?

Standing in line at a subway station the other day at 8.30 AM, I noticed the man in front of me was ranting at the woman selling tickets because he had missed his train (through no fault of hers). She had obviously been trained in people management, because she stayed calm and polite throughout and managed to calm him down. When it was my turn I commented on how well she had dealt with him and how stressful it must be. She smiled and said, *"It's the hardest part of the job. We get all sorts of people in here and most of them are fine. But some people are just so angry and because you are sitting here in the company uniform you get the full brunt of it."* Sometimes there is no one to blame when terrible things happen in our lives and the institution provides us with a scapegoat.

On some days it does seem that the whole world is against you, and the general levels of public anger are clear from all the Plexiglas windows now erected in banks and ticket offices to protect employees from the public. This is unfocused, free-floating anger waiting to settle on the nearest victim who raises his or her head above the parapet. If you happen to bump up against someone like this at the bus stop or in the lunch line and say or do the wrong thing, you are likely to witness an explosion. Sound familiar? Maybe you have even been there yourself?

But we all have contact with organizations that sometimes behave badly. We may be trying to get through the interminable spider web of a call center to change an insurance policy. Perhaps our bank has behaved badly, or we have been trying to buy a house and the real estate agents have pulled a fast one on us, or the mechanics at the local garage have done a number on us when we took the car in for a tune up. So how do we begin to come to forgiveness with an institution?

The key difficulty is that there is generally no identifiable person who has done us wrong. Often it is impossible to pin down exactly who is to blame for the error that has caused us problems. Even if we have a name, in a large organization it's unlikely that you will reach that particular individual for an apology. It is much more likely that you will have to tell your story all over again to another person. This is where displaced anger sets in—and we have all been there. We get through to an unhelpful clerk who tells us it is not their department, puts us on hold for ten minutes, then cuts us off. When we call back to rant at them, another, wholly innocent person takes the brunt of our displaced anger. Taking it out on the wrong person is clearly not the answer. If you have a genuine grievance:

- make detailed and accurate notes of what has happened;
- find out who is in charge of customer relations;
- stay calm and make it clear you are not going to give up;
- make a note of the person's name and the conversation and follow it up with a letter, detailing what action you now expect; and
- make it more worth the company's while to solve the problem and have you go away;

But often the day-to-day minutiae that needs forgiveness is not worth making a formal complaint about. It takes the wind out of our sails and can make our blood pressure rise, so how do we cope with that?

Bringing an organization into the Forgiveness Room

Go back to the Forgiveness Room. Find a symbol for the company and place it on the chair opposite you. Now take the company through the usual process, first telling your version of how much this affected you and then standing behind its chair, before getting the third perspective. Now let it go.

Letting go of the need to blame the messenger

Sometimes, we focus our anger and bitterness on the messenger of bad news. When Betty was in her late twenties, her mother was diagnosed with terminal cancer; she died a year later. Initially Betty felt very angry with the doctor who had told them the news. *"When I was first told that my mother had terminal cancer, I was in the room with her and the doctor. Looking back on it he did the best he could, he was a messenger of incredibly bad news but at the time I couldn't forgive him for telling me that. Because he told me and my mother that she was going to die, essentially, in that moment all my previous fears about hospital visits came together and I hated that doctor. Looking back on it now, I realize that he was only doing his job."*

Betty hated the fact that her mother was dying and she couldn't do anything about it. But she could hate the people who couldn't save her mother. Betty found herself blaming the doctors, then the hospital, then the world itself for her mother's death. *"I hated hospitals and the medical profession. I hated them because they couldn't do anything. They kept on saying, 'We can look after her and make her last few months comfortable'; it was symbolic of our powerlessness."*

Betty did, in the end, manage to forgive the hospital and the people caring for her mother because she came to understand that her anger and bitterness were displaced. *"In the end I forgave the institution, the palliative care nurse who said, 'Look, we can't save your mother's life but we can make her last few weeks bearable.' I hated her for saying that but in the end I came to respect her because she was doing her best and she did help a lot."*

Letting go does not mean forgetting what happened

When an organization is held accountable for the behavior of its members the forgiveness fallout can be devastating. Many people, for example, have recently come forward to talk about the abuse, both physical and sexual, they have suffered at the hands of nuns and priests in the Roman Catholic Church. Between 2002 and 2003 a total of forty-eight Catholic priests in the United States were convicted of offences against children, many of the offences dating back years. The widespread allegations of abuse and cover-up in America, England, Australia, and elsewhere have brought the Church to crisis point.

Tina was ten when she was molested by her parish priest. At the time she didn't tell anyone except a friend and it wasn't until she was seventeen that she told her mother. "*I went to a funeral and the priest was up in the pulpit. I was an angry, aggressive seventeen-year-old at the time and I just said to my mother if I had a gun, I'd blow that man's balls off. She was stunned and pretty shocked and she didn't quite believe me and I think I tried to explain to her later why. She knew I resented the Church at the time; I thought they were all a crowd of jerks. I was casting everything off then. But she was used to those endless debates that we had at home, thrashing the Church to shreds and her trying to protect it.*"

Tina never reported the incident to the police and no action has ever been taken against the priest who molested her. When I ask her if she would consider reporting him to the authorities now, she seems unsure. "*I think he's dead now . . . I'm not sure if I want to go to the police . . . I'm not sure if I would. Don't know if I would be stirring up a lot of things. I would probably have been the least abused by that priest of a lot of the kids in that community because I wasn't actively involved in the youth club. I might just be stirring up things that they choose not to be interested in. Was it such a big bad thing? He didn't have sex with me, he just manhandled me. I am incensed by it and it fucked me up in different ways and it added to the layers that caused me not to be able to respect myself, so he's hugely culpable, but the context of that community is not so important to me anymore.*"

It is very hard to rock the boat in a small community. Tina has all sorts of good reasons for not reporting the incident. Victims of sexual abuse often find themselves taking responsibility for what happened in some way, such as in Tina's case, asking whether it was such a bad thing, compared to what happened to others. But it has to be an individual decision, based on balancing many different factors. No one can tell a victim to report someone to the authorities;

it must always be the victim's choice. In the past we have seen only too often that victims were not believed, thus adding to the pain of abuse. And, of course, recognition and punishment of the offender is only a step on the road to forgiveness.

Tina is still struggling with forgiveness, though she is aware of how not coming to forgiveness hurts her. *"I certainly don't forgive him; if I could get him now I'd murder him. But that is my destructive rage that I have to accept and observe."*

And if she has not forgiven the individual who molested her, what about the organization of the Church?

"Forgiven the Church—no! I suppose I still have an awful lot of resentment in me about a lot of things and sometimes it is easier to decide that the institution is something I could kick the stuffing out of."

In such cases there are two issues—the forgiveness of the individual and of the organization that often did not act appropriately when the abuse was brought to its attention. If the organization did not respond as it should, then the organization itself needs forgiveness too. In forgiveness terms, it is possible to be as bitter with an organization as an individual; in some ways it is much easier, as an organization like a church makes a big and vulnerable target.

In this issue the Catholic Church has, broadly speaking, used the classic avoidance tactics that institutions often try and use to avoid blame, by first denying the problem existed, then suggesting that the problem was one of individual bad apples rather than a systemic problem within the organization. Such denials, of course, make forgiveness even more painful and difficult for those who have suffered. Yet individual churchmen have been brave enough to apologize. Across the United States and England, many individual priests have had the courage to ask for forgiveness for the organization that they represent from the pulpit.

Learning the lessons

If you belong to an organization or group and it has behaved in ways that you strongly disapprove of, how do you forgive the organization and remain an active member? The key to forgiveness in this situation is to remember that the organization is made up of individuals—individual human beings with their capacity for good and evil. Think of the groups you belong to:

- ethnic group
- religion
- nationality
- work
- social

Now, just for once, think of all the terrible things your groups have done throughout history or even within your own lifetime. Write them down. It doesn't make comfortable reading for any of us. What it shows us is that all groups get it very wrong sometimes. We may have had nothing to do with the serious wrong our group did to others but it may have been done in our name and we may also still collectively be blamed. Justice needs to be served, but then we need to move on.

Forgiveness allows us all to move on.

An exercise in forgiveness

Begin as always with some meditation to leave the outside world behind and get yourself to a peaceful place. Now do some life breaths.

Think of the groups you need to forgive and those from which you need forgiveness.

- What institution do you need to forgive?
- Is it your school, your bank, a religious group, another nation?
- Are you ready to forgive it? Bring it into the Forgiveness Room, using a symbol of the organization. Work through the forgiveness process and let the group go.
- Now do you need to ask forgiveness from a group?

Think carefully . . . this will be much harder. Bring them into the Forgiveness Room and work through the forgiveness process with them. Now let them go.

Beyond national boundaries

When you widen forgiveness beyond national boundaries, it can become even more difficult to keep perspective. We have only to look at the Middle East, the Balkans, Rwanda, and Northern Ireland to understand how difficult forgiveness in the wider world has become.

Yet there is increasing evidence that world leaders are beginning to recognize that forgiveness is essential to the healing of wounds, however old. From 1932 until 1972, the U.S. Public Health Service allowed more than 400 black men to go untreated for syphilis after offering them free medical care. The men were never told they were part of a study, clinically named the Tuskegee Study of Untreated Syphilis in the Negro Male, nor were they informed they had syphilis. Government doctors failed to offer the standard treatment method, mercury and arsenic, when it became available. Nor did doctors offer penicillin shots once it became the standard method of curing the disease. The men received treatment only after the experiment became public in 1972.

In 1997, sixty-five years after the U.S. Public Health Service began secret experiments on them, President Clinton apologized to five black men ranging in age from eighty-seven to one hundred and ten.

If you are serious about asking for forgiveness there can be no ifs and buts. It is hard to acknowledge that you are completely in the wrong, particularly when you are apologizing on behalf of a nation. But President Clinton did just that. *"The United States Government did something that was wrong, deeply, profoundly, morally wrong. It was an outrage to our commitment to integrity and equality for all our citizens. We can end the silence. We can stop turning our heads away. We can look you in the eye and finally say on behalf of the American people what the United States Government did was shameful, and I am sorry."* [6]

By that time, twenty-eight men had died of syphilis, a hundred others were dead of related complications, forty wives and nineteen children had been infected. The government a few years later paid the survivors and relatives ten million dollars in damages but without a formal apology.

Clinton also said, *"Today all we can do is apologize, but ... only you have the power to forgive. Your presence here shows us that you have chosen a better path than your government did so long ago. You have not withheld the power to forgive. What was done cannot be undone, but we can end the silence."*

Nations have also realized the importance of asking forgiveness of those they have wronged in their own country. In Australia a national "Sorry Day" was held on May 26, 1998, exactly a year after the tabling in the Federal Parliament of the report of the National

Inquiry into the removal of Aboriginal and Torres Strait Islander children from their families.

The report, "Bringing Them Home," revealed the extent of forced removal, which went on for 150 years and its consequences in terms of broken families, shattered physical and mental health, loss of language, culture, and connection to traditional land, loss of parenting skills, and the enormous distress of many of its victims today.

The purpose of the semi-official "National Sorry Day" organized in Australia, sponsored by various government agencies, state and local administrations, and churches and business leaders, was for the "nation" to apologize to the Aboriginal people for the forced removal of more than 100,000 children from their families between the 1880s and 1960s.

The campaign won the sympathy of wide layers of professional and working people, reflected in the collection of one million signatures and handwritten messages in "Sorry Books."

In 2002 a community initiative was launched to support all who suffer as a result of the removal policies; called "The Journey of Healing," it was conceived by members of the so-called "stolen generations" (of Aboriginal children) in response to the 1998 national Sorry Day. *"If healing is to come, Indigenous and non-Indigenous must work for it together. Everyone can find the next step toward healing, but may need help. The Journey offers every Australian the chance to help.*

A million Australians have shown their longing for reconciliation through Sorry Books and bridge walks. This year we offer everyone the chance to take a further step toward justice and healing." [7]

The strength of the Journey of Healing initiative is that it recognizes that forgiveness is a process. Saying sorry is crucial. But it is a step in the process. It is not enough to just say sorry; forgiveness requires repentance and reparation and time. Wounds take a long time to heal and scars are always visible. Often the offender believes that it is enough to apologize, that the slate is immediately and permanently wiped clean. But forgiveness does not work like that. It involves a change in the heart and spirit, first to make sure that the offence could never happen again, then to deal with the fallout of what has been done. For true forgiveness to take place both sides have to let go. In a situation like that faced by the Australian nation, that freedom is a long journey of trust.

Are you willing to let go of being part of the problem and become part of the solution?

Begin as always with some meditation to leave the outside world behind and get yourself to a peaceful place. Now do some life breaths.

How are you doing with forgiveness? Are you at peace with yourself, your neighbor, your family? Take yourself to the Forgiveness Room and rest there in peace for a while.

Try repeating the Jain mantra: *"I seek forgiveness from all beings, I offer forgiveness to all beings. All beings are my friends. I have no enemies."*

Now imagine your peaceful, loving spirit as a beautiful smooth stone. This is your peaceful harmonious wish for the world, that it should be filled with love and tenderness and forgiveness. Look at your stone, hold it in your hand, feel how smooth it is. Maybe it is warm from the sun. As you hold it in your hand fill it with all your wishes for peace in the world; fill it with attentive forgiveness.

Now imagine yourself in a boat in the middle of a lake. The water is so calm there is not a ripple. Can you see the edge of the lake? What is it like? Maybe there is a forest running down to the edge; you might catch a glimpse of a deer coming down to drink.

Now take your stone, full of your wishes for peace and forgiveness, and drop it into the middle of the lake. The water is very clear; you'll be able to watch the stone sinking through the water. Watch the ripples as they fan out from the boat, moving outward into the world. These are your hopes and wishes for peace and forgiveness in the world.

Letting go of our fear of the other

Where there is fear of the other, forgiveness cannot work. To feel comfortable in our own identity we first distinguish and identify the other as "not us." Then comes the isolation and hostility. History has shown us tragically and graphically how the identification of the other can lead to genocide. Watch the news—any breakdown of peace is predicated on the identification of the other. But why is our own identity so dependent on the identification of the other? If I am a man and you are a woman, if I am a Jew and you are a Muslim, if I am black and you are white, must we be defined simply in opposition to one another? Do I not exist as a man if you are not a woman?

Environmentalist and peace campaigner Satish Kumar made a two-and-a-half-year walk for peace that took him to the capital cities of the nuclear powers to deliver a message of peace to their leaders. His journey began symbolically at Mahatma Gandhi's grave in India and ended at John F. Kennedy's grave in Arlington National Cemetery. On leaving India he headed for the Pakistan border. A friend wanted to give him enough food and water to last him through the journey through "hostile territory," as Pakistan is a nation that is upheld as the great enemy of India. Satish Kumar thanked him for his compassion in offering him provisions but refused to accept the "packets of mistrust." "*If you travel as a pilgrim, you will meet other pilgrims.*" He found a warm welcome throughout his trip through enemy country.

One of the things he realized on his walk across the world for peace is that leaders are so often caught up in *realpolitik* that they bypass ordinary human reactions.

"So the force and the strength for peace will come from people. And deep down we share the same humanity, the global humanity. That's what I experienced. I went through so many different cultures—Muslim, Jewish, Christian, Hindu, Buddhist, Russian, American, European, Asian, Black, White, Brown, Socialist, Communist— you name them and I met them. And when you dig down, dig deep, and touch the humanity, they are the same everywhere. But before you can discover that unity, you have to be free of your own prejudices. Because if I went as an Indian waving the flag of India, I would meet a Pakistani. If I went as a Hindu, saying that Hinduism is the most supreme religion in the world, I would meet a Christian or a Muslim saying, 'No, no, no! You've got it wrong. We have got the best religion.' If I go as a Socialist I'll meet a Capitalist. If I go as a brown man I'll meet a black man or white man. But if I go as a human being I'll meet only human beings." [8]

If we recognize our interdependence the building of walls becomes nonsensical. If we are one, why would I wish to harm you? If you can understand my wish not to harm you, why would you want to harm me? Forgiveness turns the equation of fear on its head. If I replace fear, which is at the basis of all hatred between communities, with forgiveness, whom shall I fear?

Notes

[1] Tutu, Desmond, *No Future Without Forgiveness*, (Rider, 1999), p. 107

[2] Ibid, p. 28

[3] Ibid, p. 129

[4] Ibid, p. 127

[5] Kübler-Ross, Elisabeth, and Kessler, David, *Life Lessons: Two Experts on Death and Dying Teach Us About the Mysteries of Life and Living* (Simon & Schuster, 2000)

[6] President Clinton, in a speech on 16 May 1997

[7] See the excellent Web sites www.reconciliationaustralia.org and www.journeyofhealing.com

[8] Satish Kumar, The Forgiveness Conference, 18 October 1999, The Findhorn Foundation

8

Forgive
and Remember

O Lord, remember not only the men and women of good will,
But also those of evil will.
And in remembering the suffering they inflicted upon us;
Honour the fruits we have borne thanks to this suffering—
Our comradeship, our humility, our compassion,
Our courage, our generosity, the greatness of heart
Which has grown out of all this;
And when they come to the judgement,
Let all the fruits that we have borne,
Be their forgiveness . . .

ANY PEOPLE MAKE the mistake of thinking that to forgive is to forget. That what has been done somehow needs to be blanked from the memory. Yet the whole of our functioning lives as human beings is based on our ability to remember things. We learn by remembering. As babies we are taught by repeating things over and over again; it's how we acquire language, the idea of how the world works—hot things burn, water makes us wet, this made us happy last time we did it, this person is mother. . . . crawling, then standing on our own two feet.

"To forget": from the Old English fogietan, meaning to lose from the mind, be unable to remember, or to leave behind by mistake.

"To remember": from the Latin re + memorare, meaning to bring to mind.

If we forgive and forget, we do just that—leave behind by mistake, rather than learning from our experience. So what is the purpose of remembering?

Think of the last new skill that you learned: how did you learn it? By memorizing and repetition. Learning a new language or learning to drive, or how to cook a complex dish. You learn the basics and then you repeat them until you know them so well that you don't have to think about them.

Now think of your best memory; it might be

- A sunlit meal with friends
- A special moment with children
- Recognizing you were in love
- Swimming in a beautiful place

Spend some time going over the memory, taking yourself through the whole experience. Feel how real it is to you; can you almost smell and touch it? What did you learn from it?

Now do the same with your worst memory; it might be

- A terrible fight
- The breakup of a relationship

- The death of someone close to you
- An illness

Spend some time with this memory; take yourself through the whole experience. Feel how real it is; what did you learn from it?

It's clear from these two exercises that memory, the act of "bringing things to mind," is crucial in our lives. And memory is just as vital when it comes to forgiveness.

Gone but not forgotten

When we say "I forgot" it's generally negative—we use it as an excuse for missed appointments, or things we should have done. Forgiveness is no different. Letting go means that the bitterness has really gone, but forgetting allows the bad stuff to happen again.

Remembering is not the same as being stuck.

Before we come to forgiveness our painful memories keep us stuck in the past. We can go over and over the events in our lives, never moving forward or allowing them to change. Remembering the past and dealing with it allows us to let it go while learning the lessons we have to learn. The remembering has a purpose beyond the simple recall of events. Otherwise we fall into a sort of forgiveness amnesia.

Amnesia: from the Greek *a* + *mnasthai*, meaning not to remember.

In some countries where human rights had been violated, like Chile, the leaders and perpetrators made amnesty a condition of handing over power. So Pinochet and his government effectively forgave themselves with a blanket amnesty. Of course, that did not stop the stories being told, but the lack of official recognition makes it impossible to have a sense of justice and therefore forgiveness is officially frozen. Amnesty becomes amnesia.

Forgetting means burying the past; remembering allows us to honor the past, as individuals in our own lives, as beings with a sense of history.

As individuals this means that when we come up against situations that have hurt us in the past, we can "bring them to mind" and act accordingly.

As beings with a sense of history, we can make sure that the most terrible acts of violence are not forgotten so that we do not repeat them.

How does remembering help in forgiveness?

- ❧ It allows us to learn from the past.
- ❧ It allows us to change the future.
- ❧ It allows us to stop whatever happened from happening again.

Is everything forgivable?

If we are to learn from the past, in our individual histories or as human beings, we have to remember and let go. Does forgiveness mean that everything is forgivable? It is only in acknowledging our own capacity for hatred that forgiveness stands a chance in our own lives or internationally.

The last decade of the twentieth century showed that the human race still had a long way to go. It seemed that a bloodthirsty century finished in a crescendo of violence. The massacres in Rwanda and the Balkans, to name but two areas of the world, astonished us by their ferocity.

As we move into our new millennium, there are plenty of examples only too fresh in our memories that seem to stand outside any possibility of forgiveness.

On August 15, 1998, at 3.10 PM, in the middle of a busy Saturday afternoon's shopping, terrorists set off a bomb in the middle of Omagh in Northern Ireland. It was the single worst incident in Northern Ireland in the current conflict. Twenty-nine people were killed and hundreds were injured, including several children.

All the losses were appalling, but one family, the Grimes, was particularly hard hit. Mick Grimes lost his wife, Mary (it was her sixty-fifth birthday), his thirty-year-old daughter, Avril Monaghan, and his eighteen-month-old granddaughter, Maura, who was the youngest victim. Avril was seven months pregnant with twins and they died in the atrocity too.

It is difficult to understand how people could plant a bomb in the middle of a busy Saturday afternoon, knowing that dozens of people were likely to be killed. The very idea of forgiveness seems inappropriate, unimaginable. Surely this act must be outside the bounds of forgiveness? Again it is in the darkest episodes of our history that the answer to the question of whether everything is forgivable will be found.

A desire for revenge would seem to be the natural reaction in such circumstances. Yet when we read Mick Grimes's account of his reactions (and remember he lost his wife, daughter, granddaughter, and unborn twin grandchildren) something different is going on.

"Mary had gone to town with our daughter Avril and eighteen-month-old grand-daughter Maura to do some shopping for the birth of Avril's twins in a few weeks' time. I was the only one at home—it was a reasonably good summer's day, a holiday

as far as we were concerned. I heard the explosion, but I didn't know where the sound came from.

Some of our children had sent their mother a big bouquet for her birthday. Minutes after I heard the explosion, an Interflora man came to deliver the bouquet. He'd heard it, too, and we talked about what the explosion might be. He said he thought it was in Omagh.

It wasn't until the next morning that we heard that one of those killed was a pregnant mother. We thought that must be Avril. Then we knew that she and Mary, my wife, would all have been close together.

Later we learned that they had been in the draper's shop buying some material for clothes. After they'd bought what they wanted, Avril had lifted up Maura into her arms and the little girl had waved "bye bye" to everyone in the shop. "She was so lovely, everyone smiled and laughed," the shop assistant who survived the bomb told us. Moments later, all three had left the shop, and were killed.

There was no trouble in identifying Maura because she was so little, the youngest victim. Later on my sons were asked to identify Avril because she had been so badly burned. They had to use fingerprint tests to identify my wife. My other daughter's baby was born the day after the funeral.

My loss is great: my wife, my daughter, my granddaughter. And today there should have been the twins, my two little granddaughters who would have been ten-and-a-half months old.

The police told us they would catch the people responsible for Omagh. I said, "Don't seek vengeance on our account. That's not going to get us anywhere." Tit for tat is like children quarrelling; it's fruitless.

For me this has been a hard and lonely year. I've had many changes in my life. Too many changes. Our loss has left two houses without a woman, without a mother.

I am a Catholic but there is no difference between my Protestant neighbor and the one up the road who is a Catholic. On this anniversary I'd like to ask the politicians to listen to the vast majority of people in Northern Ireland who long for peace. And to live in this part of the world in peace would be heaven."[1]

If Mick Grimes can plead for peace, where does that leave the rest of us in forgiveness? It seems he has instinctively understood something vital about the process: that justice must be served, of course; but that vengeance is not an option. It would only mean another family grieving somewhere else.

More importantly, his view is that we are all one. That the differences between Protestant and Catholic mean nothing in the face of such suffering; any decent member of either community would have the same reaction.

If we look at the terrible events of the last century—the two world wars, the Holocaust, Rwanda, Kosovo, South Africa, Northern Ireland—it seems that some things must remain unforgivable. Yet it is at precisely this moment of agony that the very heart of forgiveness lies. It is in the darkness of these terrible acts that we can come closer to understanding how the process of forgiveness works.

Hatred on a group level

In the deliberate use of such violence, the terror comes from being a target as part of a group—Catholic, Protestant, Jew, Tutsi. When you are chosen because you belong to a group that has been identified as the enemy, you lose your individuality in the sight of the attacker. You are not singled out for anything you have done or the sort of person you are, but for simply being other. And at that point both the attacker and the victim lose what makes us essentially human—our uniqueness.

That identification with the group continues to operate when we don't forgive. Hatred and bitterness work on the group level. A survivor of the extermination camps may well spend his or her life hating all Germans, or a Tutsi may just wait for revenge against the

Hutu tribe who massacred his or her family and his village. But if the Balkans have taught us anything, it is that sustained group hatred can only lead to more revenge and bloodshed. And that bitterness can be nurtured for generations.

While the different ethnic communities in former Yugoslavia lived next to each other in peace for many years, it was still possible for the Serbs to slit the throats of their neighbors, to shoot their children and rape their daughters as though they no longer knew them. In a terrible way, they didn't; each individual had lost the tag that makes him or her special, human, and precious. In becoming identified with a hated group they had lost their individuality and by losing their individuality they had ceased to be human.

This was only too clearly demonstrated by the way the Serbs tore up the identity cards of the Albanians they came across—if you don't have a name you are no longer an individual and you don't matter.

Mick Grimes understands at a profound level that hating an individual who happens to belong to the group that planted the bomb resolves nothing. They were no more responsible for the bomb than he was. He manages, somehow, to see the "other side" as a group of individuals, each to be judged on his or her own separate merit, not identified merely as group members.

The Omagh bomb turned out to have been planted by the Real IRA, so ironically, by the "Catholic" side. This makes hating the individuals who belong to the group that perpetrate an atrocity all the more ironic—for how do you hate your own side? Yourself?

Letting go of needing an enemy

In her book *Friends and Enemies* Dorothy Rowe explains how enemies can serve a useful function. *"Most of us have in childhood the kind of experiences which* lead us to believe that we are not good enough as we are. Any person who can assure us merely by their existence that we are acceptable becomes very precious to us. Hence enemies become very precious. Some people keep a stock of enemies and arrange them in a hierarchy so that they have always got someone to feel superior to." [2]

In this context enemies become a necessity, a way of defining who we are and who we are not. After visiting the Serbian command post in the village of Mirkovci in Croatia during the Serbo-Croat war in 1993, Michael Ignatieff pointed out in his book *The Warrior's Honor* that not only do we identify the individual enemy as a member of a group, but we lose our own individual definition, and at that moment lose something of our humanity. "*The kind of Serb this man believes himself to have been before the war is not the kind of Serb he became after the war. Before the war, he might have thought of himself as a Yugoslav or café manager or a husband rather than as a Serb. Now as he sits in this farmhouse bunker, there are men two hundred and fifty yards away who would kill him. For them he is only a Serb, not a neighbor, not a friend, not a Yugoslav, not a former team mate at the football club. And because he is only a Serb for his enemies, he has become only a Serb to himself.*" [3]

If we are not defined first by our humanity we are lost. Once you become "only a Serb," "only a Hutu," or "only a Jew," any atrocity is possible.

You may think that you are not caught up by this sort of thinking. Try answering these questions:

- What do these words bring to mind: Democrat, Republican, Green Party Member, Evangelical Christian?
- What about these words: feminist, man, woman, homosexual?
- Can you name a group you dislike?

While we can all remember incidents when we have been the victims, it is much more uncomfortable to acknowledge when we have been on the side of prejudice and ignorance. As a feminist I have often caught myself lumping all men together as the oppressor—and that is just lazy thinking. Or in the office dismissing anyone in the higher ranks as a suit—disregarding their individual human worth. Although a convenient shorthand, it is too easy to dismiss the sort of person we dislike as being part of a group. Once they become just a part of a group they lose what makes them essentially human—their individuality.

Tribal reactions—the hatred of the other—are not a conscious choice on our parts. But deciding to look at our most uncomfortable tribal feelings is essential to forgiveness. One by one we can make a difference, by ensuring that we do not fall into the group psychosis or that when we do, we examine it clearly and own up to feelings, however difficult they may be. And to do that we need to realize and admit that those feelings are not necessarily of our own making but that the group psychosis has been handed down to us through the generations.

How to free ourselves of tribal thinking

We are all tribal. Believe you are immune from tribal thinking? Take a minute to define yourself:

- man/woman
- gay/straight
- nationality
- political party
- religious faith

Pretty quickly you will find a group comes to mind that you make jokes about, dislike, could even hate if pushed. Though most of us, thankfully, will never experience the terrible events in Northern Ireland or Kosovo or Rwanda, we are all nevertheless tribal, with a strong capacity for hatred.

As a Catholic living in Liverpool, U.K., when I see Protestant Orangemen with their uniforms and bands trying to march down the Roman Catholic Garvahey Road in Northern Ireland to provoke violence, I am enraged. But it is not just Kathleen the individual who is enraged; she has the history of generations of Catholics who have been oppressed in Northern Ireland standing behind her. I feel rage and hatred against the Orangemen even though none of them has ever done anything to me personally. But in identifying with the group, I feel the group hatred. It is tribal—just as they have lost their individuality, so I have lost mine. We have both become no more than members of our tribe. What is perhaps more surprising, more difficult to admit, is that in many ways it is a comfortable feeling. I don't have to think or individualize; just see the man in the bowler hat with the furled umbrella and the appropriate group feeling of hatred arises. The tribal images are so strongly pro-grammed within us that we stop behaving and thinking like an individual as we would normally.

I can now belong to a group that gives me an instant identity—and one that is even more comfortable in that it takes the side of the wronged and dispossessed. I have divided the world into them and us, with reason on my side alone.

Who is the other for you?

When that feeling is reflected back at me from the other side, we become like two mirrors reflecting the heat of our hatred more and more fiercely until we are both consumed. That is also why any fraternization with the enemy is seen as betrayal and why any attempt at friendliness or intermarriage is seen as threatening and the offenders are killed. However, if Romeo and Juliet not only love each other but manage to set aside the traditional hatred to make a life together, then the group hatred will melt away, for both communities will understand that the other is in fact much like themselves—the same mix of humanity.

If we belong to a minority group, we will often have been picked on and that will have brought us into the fold of group safety more tightly. But it will rarely have led us to question whether our very belonging to a certain group has made us pick on others. It is only when we understand that the tribal prejudices we condemn in others are also very much present in ourselves that there is any hope for forgiveness and peace in the world.

At a conference on forgiveness held in Findhorn in 1999 I was shown this starkly and most uncomfortably myself. Colin Craig, the director of the Corrymeela community in Northern Ireland, had given a moving talk about his work in the community. Corrymeela has been set up as a reconciliation center between the two communities of Protestants and Roman Catholics. They have worked with everyone in the community including children, teachers, and paramilitaries. [4]

They quickly realized that the first essential step was to get the communities to physically meet in the same room. Even teachers in Northern Ireland could go through their whole lives without meeting someone from the other community in any normal setting. As children they would go to Catholic or Protestant schools, live in Catholic or Protestant areas, go to Catholic or Protestant teacher training college, and then back into a Catholic or Protestant school for the remainder of their working lives. Without ever having had to meet someone from the other community, fear and fantasy could thrive.

Colin Craig then held a workshop on reconciliation around the issues in Northern Ireland. His view is that we need to be encouraged to reveal our humanity to one another. *"The challenge is to facilitate ways in which people can begin to see beyond the messages and 'the story' that automatically comes into play as soon as the 'other' is labeled as a Catholic or Protestant."*

There were about twenty of us at the workshop. First he got us into same-faith groups and asked us to come up with *"What is the question that you have always wanted to ask the other?"* When we came together we read them out and were shocked to discover that they were almost identical. "We" both had more or less the same questions to ask "them."

After a break for coffee we found we knew exactly who belonged to what group; effectively all of us in the room knew precisely who "the enemy" was. Although we were in no danger from anyone, we had all memorized who was on "our side"—though none of us had ever met before. And in a workshop where everyone was either working on or interested in forgiveness, we could identify the enemy and be prepared for whatever they might do.

The facilitator then said, *"Now take away your education and your willingness to be involved in forgiveness and pretend that each of you has a machine gun."*

He spent the rest of the morning getting us to mix and experience each other as individuals through various exercises and games. It was an extremely uncomfortable time for everyone. Here we were, "forgiveness professionals," being confronted with very stark and primitive prejudices against people we had never met and yet were prepared to label without hesitation.

It was deeply uncomfortable for us to acknowledge how we, an educated, liberal group who thought forgiveness a peachy idea, were at heart deeply tribal and prejudiced. So the hatred wasn't just out there in the world but firmly implanted and flowering nicely within our own hearts. It is only when we can recognize our own capacity for hatred that forgiveness stands a chance.

> History, despite its wrenching pain
> Cannot be unlived, but if faced with courage
> Need not be lived again
>
> MAYA ANGELOU

Remembering the lessons of history

If forgiveness has any value, it must be indivisible. So it follows that everything, theoretically, must be forgivable. Yet surely there must be some events that should stand outside the normal parameters of forgiveness? Genocide is the obvious example—the deliberate attempt at extermination of a whole nation or group. The Holocaust has often been quoted as an event that must stand outside normal parameters of forgiveness because of the special quality of evil perpetrated against the Jews.

Simon Wiesenthal asks this very question in relation to the Holocaust. His Dokumentationscentrum, which seeks out Nazi criminals, has helped to bring over 1100 Nazis to justice since the end of the war.

He himself is a survivor of the extermination camps and during his time there was involved in a case that presented him with a moral dilemma. He confronts us with the same dilemma fifty years on.

In the book *The Sunflower* he describes how, when he was in an extermination camp, he was sent out on a work detail. At the local hospital he was taken by a nurse to a figure on a bed in a room by himself. *"Now I could see the figure in the bed far more clearly. White, bloodless hands on the counterpane, head completely bandaged with openings only for mouth, nose, and ears."* [5]

The figure on the bed, Karl, had joined the SS as a volunteer. He was from Stuttgart and was twenty-one years old. He knew he was dying and wanted to confess his crime and be forgiven. He had taken part in a massacre, pushing three hundred Jews—men, women, and children—into a house, dousing it with gasoline, and throwing hand grenades into it. A father carrying a little boy and a mother had jumped from the window rather than be burnt to death and it was that image that had stayed with Karl.

"The pains in my body are terrible, but worse still is my conscience. It never ceases to remind me of the burning house and family that jumped from the window" [6]

Wiesenthal says, *"In his confession there was true repentance, even though he did not admit it in so many words. Nor was it necessary, for the way he spoke and the fact that he spoke to me was a proof of his repentance.* [7]

Karl said, 'I do not know who you are, I only know that you are a Jew and that is enough. I want to die in peace, and so I need' . . . I saw that he could not get the words past his lips. But I was in no mood to help him. I kept silent. 'I know that what I have told you is terrible. In the long nights while I have been waiting for death, time and time again I have longed to talk about it to a Jew and beg forgiveness from him. Only I didn't know whether there were any Jews left . . . I know that what I am asking is almost too much for you, but without your answer I cannot die in peace.'"

Simon Wiesenthal was sure that the man was dying and equally sure that he himself would not survive the extermination camp for much longer.

"Here lay a man in bed who wished to die in peace—but he could not, because the memory of his terrible crime gave him no rest. And by him sat a man also doomed

to die—but who did not want to die because he yearned to see the end of all the horror that blighted the world."

Simon Wiesenthal left the room without a word and refused to forgive the man. He wondered if he had done the right thing and back in the camp he talked to his friends and one of them, Josek, said, "I feared at first, that you had really forgiven him. You would have had no right to do this in the name of people who had not authorized you to do so. What people have done to you yourself, you can, if you like, forgive and forget. That is your own affair. But it would have been a terrible sin to burden your conscience with other people's sufferings. You have suffered nothing because of him, and it follows that what he has done to other people you are in no position to forgive."[8] Josek did not survive the war.

There is an additional twist to the story. Wiesenthal met Karl's mother after the war and she thought of her son as a hero. Wiesenthal chose not to reveal what her son had done.

What would you have done?

In *The Sunflower*, Simon Wiesenthal asks different writers and philosophers what they would have done in the circumstances. By implication he puts the same question to us readers. His own view is clear: "The crux of the matter is, of course, the question of forgiveness. Forgetting is something that time alone takes care of, but forgiveness is an act of volition, and only the sufferer is qualified to make the decision."

One of those writers consulted, Alan L. Berger, also made another important point: "In asking a Jew to hear his confession, Karl perpetuated the Nazi stereotype. Jews were not individuals with souls, feelings, aspirations, and emotions. Rather, they were perceived as an amorphous, undifferentiated mass. Bring me a Jew, was the dying Nazi's request. Any Jew will do."[9]

Harold S. Kushner, Rabbi laureate of Temple Israel in Natick, understands that forgiveness is an individual matter of conscience and that because we forgive certainly does not mean we condone or forget what has happened.

"Forgiving happens inside us. It represents a letting go of the sense of grievance, and perhaps most importantly a letting go of the role of victim. For a Jew to forgive the Nazis would not mean, God forbid, saying to them, 'What you did was understandable, I can understand what led you to do it and I don't hate you for it.' It would mean saying, 'What you did was thoroughly despicable and puts you outside the category of decent human beings. But I refuse to give you the power to define me as a victim. I refuse to let your blind hatred define the shape and content of my Jewishness. I don't hate you; I reject you. And then the Nazi would remain chained to his past and to his conscience, but the Jew would be free.'"

Leaving the past behind to live in the future . . .

If forgiveness is to have any meaning at all, it must be on the individual level, one to one. Whatever I have been through, it is not for me to tell you how you must forgive. Whatever you have experienced, you cannot tell me how I must forgive. We all travel our own journey of forgiveness. What we do know is that people who have had these experiences have come to forgiveness. That it is possible.

The problem with not being able to forgive is that it doesn't stop with the individual who has caused us harm—particularly in cases of genocide. The idea of collective guilt is one that is still argued by many of those unable to forgive. In this argument, all Germans, even those born since the Holocaust, have a collective and ongoing responsibility and guilt for the atrocities committed by that generation.

While we must reject the idea of collective guilt, because people who were not born at the time of the Holocaust cannot be held responsible, is repentance alone enough? And surely repentance is a process requiring some restoration—saying sorry is not enough. What happens when all those involved are dead? So understandably some survivors of the camps have found it impossible to forgive Germans or Germany. But this leads to difficult questions of responsibility. Thus the extermination camp victim has an undeniable case for bitterness and justice against the prison guard at Dachau. The case is also undeniable against those who supported and set up the camp, those who supported the regime.

- But what of those who tried to help, who actively opposed the regime?
- Or those who were themselves, though German, persecuted?
- Or subsequent generations of Germans as yet unborn, whose grandfathers may have been wicked?
- And what of the camp survivor's grandson, who meets the guard's grandson—must they also hate one another?

Josek was right. We cannot forgive on behalf of others. It is not for those of us who have not suffered such traumatic events to judge or even tell the victims how they should act. Mick Grimes and others like him simply show us that light is possible in the middle of such darkness.

Simon Wiesenthal chose not to forgive in the name of others. He has spent his life bringing Nazis to justice, giving a voice to the millions who were murdered. Now when the perpetrators are in their eighties, some people say that they should be left in peace rather than dragged through the courts and put in prison. But how can we put a time limit on justice, on being held accountable?

The fear is that if we forgive we will also forget, and that will mean that we are disrespectful to the memory of those who died and that such atrocities can happen again.

The key is to forgive and remember. Forgive and honor the dead, bring the perpetrators to justice and do not forget.

Marietta Jaeger's daughter Susie was abducted in June 1973 at the age of seven during a family camping trip in Montana. For more than a year afterward, the family knew nothing of her whereabouts. Eventually a man was arrested—he had previously phoned to taunt them. Susie's body was found and Marietta Jaeger met her daughter's murderer and told him she forgave him. This is how she described her journey of forgiveness,

"I had finally come to believe that real justice is not punishment but restoration, not necessarily to how things used to be, but to how they really should be.

Though he was liable for the death penalty, I felt it would violate and profane the goodness, sweetness, and beauty of Susie's life by killing the kidnapper in her name. She was deserving of a more noble and beautiful memorial than a cold-blooded, premeditated, state-sanctioned killing of a restrained defenseless man, however deserving of death he may be deemed to be. I felt I far better honored her, not by becoming that which I deplored, but by saying that all life is sacred and worthy of preservation. So I asked the prosecutor to offer the alternative sentence for this crime, mandatory life imprisonment with no chance of parole. My request was honored, and when the alternative was offered, only then did he confess to Susie's death and also to the taking of three other young lives."

Moving on from feelings of revenge

Father Michael Lapsley believes that forgiveness requires certain conditions.

"Reparation and restitution must be integral parts of the journey of forgiveness. Forgiveness is not simply saying you're sorry, then making reparation and restitution. Are we supposed to forgive and forget the past? I want to suggest to you that all the great faith traditions of the world are remembering religions. To name three of them, what is it that on Friday, Saturday, and Sunday Muslims, Jews, and Christians are about? What are they about? Week by week, by week, by week, year in and year out. Again in my Christian faith tradition, of key importance, memory is redemptive memory. Life which comes out of death, good which comes out of evil. There is no good remembering if the memory simply keeps hatred alive; the question . . . is how do we get the poison out? How do we lay to rest that in the past which would destroy us and take from us the part which is life giving? For some it is a question of forgiveness, for everybody there is a question of how do we deal with the past? How do we heal the wounds? How do we heal our memories?"

Initially Marietta Jaeger reacted as most of us would, faced by the abduction and murder of her daughter. However, along her path of forgiveness, she sensed that she needed to move on from the natural feelings of revenge.

"Though I readily admit that initially I wanted to kill this man with my bare hands, by the time of the resolution of his crimes, I was convinced that my best and healthiest option was to forgive. In the twenty years since losing my daughter, I have been working with victims and their families, and my experience has been consistently confirmed. Victim families have every right initially to the normal, valid, human response of rage, but those persons who retain a vindictive mind-set ultimately give the offender another victim. Embittered, tormented, enslaved by the past, their quality of life is diminished. However justified, our unforgiveness undoes us. Anger, hatred, resentment, bitterness, revenge—they are death-dealing spirits, and they will 'take our lives' *on some level as surely as Susie's life was taken. I believe the only way we can be whole, healthy, happy persons is to learn to forgive. Though I would never have chosen it so, the first person to receive a gift of life from the death of my daughter . . . was me."*[10]

Think back to the worst thing that has been done to you, the action that still leaves you thirsting for revenge. Now ask yourself these questions:

- How would it feel to let go of the need for revenge?
- What would revenge bring me?
- Can I let go of the hope of the past being different?

We often hold on to our need to get even, to wipe out the terrible thing that was done to us by an action that will hurt that person just as much. But it is our pain we have to deal with. That is why we need to let go of the hope of the past being different. What happened has happened. That does not mean it was right or should have happened to you. But are you going to be defined by that moment? Or are you willing to move on?

Moving on means bringing the person into the Forgiveness Room and working through all the feelings of hatred and revenge.

Marie Deans is the founder of Murder Victims' Families for Reconciliation, which was founded in 1976 as a national organization of family members who oppose the death penalty in all cases. They also advocate programs and policies that reduce the rate of homicide and promote crime prevention and alternatives to violence.[11]

"After a murder, victims' families face two things: a death and a crime. At these times, families need help to cope with their grief and loss, and support to heal their hearts and rebuild their lives. From experience, we know that revenge is not the answer. The answer lies in reducing violence, not causing more death. The answer lies in supporting those who grieve for their lost loved ones, not creating more grieving families.

It is time we break the cycle of violence. To those who say society must take a life for a life, we say: 'Not in our name.'"

Most surprisingly of all, Murder Victims' Families for Reconciliation includes the families of those executed in its membership and has done so from the beginning. Reconciliation means leaving the past behind and constructing a different future that is not based on hatred and violence.

Learning the lessons of our own personal history

Just as history teaches us that we must look back and learn the lessons of hatred, if we are to move forward and live in a different world, where massacres and atrocities are not the answer, or even part of the question; so it is with our own lives. If we can forgive and remember, we will not have to travel that particular journey of learning again. Until we can do that—forgive and remember—we will be stuck in our past history and unable to move on.

But to forgive and remember does not mean that you are a victim; it does not mean that you allow any similar behavior to be repeated in your life.

- What would you do if your partner were unfaithful?
- What would you do if you discovered your child was shoplifting?
- What would you do if a friend stole some money from you?

The difficulty in these situations is that we often equate forgiveness with carrying on with the status quo. Some damage has been caused to the relationship, it is repaired and then you carry on as before, "as though nothing happened." Forgiveness becomes a one-time deal, with no further consequences.

But actions must have consequences.

Forgiveness is not passive. It is not simply an access-all-areas pass to bad behavior in the future. It is not about being a victim. Sometimes forgiveness becomes twisted in a relationship and the person forgives in an inappropriate way that allows the behavior to continue. Forgive and remember is the real key to future happiness.

Where are your boundaries?

Debbie met George when she had recently been made a widow; the next two years saw George beat her up, steal from her, and have affairs with other women. He lied to her constantly about where he was and who with; in fact he seemed to lie by instinct about things that didn't need to be lied about, like his age and where he had worked.

One summer George invited another woman to come and stay in "his" house and marry him, but Debbie intercepted the call accidentally. Both women were shocked, since they had vaguely met socially.

She then let him borrow a lot of money and her car . . . and he disappeared for a week, leaving her completely frantic. Eventually he phoned her and asked to meet her. She got someone else to drive her there and when they met he said he was in love with the other woman and wanted to borrow some more money and keep the car. Debbie gave him some more money but took the car back. A week later he phoned, begging to come home, saying it had all been a terrible mistake. It later transpired that both George and the other woman had conned each other into believing that they were both rich when in fact they were both penniless.

Debbie took him back and they have been living on the edge of drama ever since. "It's all right—I've hidden my jewelry . . ." is how she sums up the relationship.

Her friends began by trying to help her but after so many examples of her "forgiving" him, taking him back, they despair of any change and feel that they are watching a slow-motion car crash.

At some level George is testing Debbie out, desperate for some moral boundaries that he has never been given. "This far and no further" has no meaning for him, because he can always push the envelope back without any fear of reprisal; he will always be forgiven with no consequences.

When he has done some dramatic wrong, paradoxically the power shifts in the relationship and she is in the driving seat again, keeping him on his toes. Will she take him back or throw him out?

It is too easy to see him as a prince of darkness figure; what has happened to make him like that and how far does she encourage that side of him in order not to look at that side of herself? In other words, he gets to play the role of the bad guy, which makes her into the victim—and she gets to look good.

Forgiveness has nothing to do with passivity, with letting people trample on you until there is nothing left. Real forgiveness would involve letting him go, never allowing him to hurt her again. But then she would have to forgive herself as well and examine her own fear of being alone.

Debbie's story is dramatic, but we all come across examples in our lives where someone hurts us over and over again until we get the message and put a stop to it. Until we learn the lesson of our own history.

- How many times does this have to be done to you before you learn the lesson you are being taught?
- Do you still want to be in this situation this time next year? In ten years' time?
- Are you willing to stop connecting in this way?
- What is your "crunch point"—this far and no further?

Stopping the abusive behavior is the first step in the forgiveness process.

Debbie needs to understand a valuable lesson: George will never change; he will always let her down. She needs to say no to his abusive behavior and just have it stop. Usually you have to stop the behavior and get out of the line of fire before you can begin to embark on the path of forgiveness. To forgive and remember is to avoid falling into the trap of "If I have forgiven you, it means you won't do it again." So forgive the behavior, but don't let yourself be exploited again.

Cutting the connection of hatred

I believe that it only takes one person to begin the process, to cut the connection of hatred. The human race has not yet learned the lessons of history. We are still tribal, still hate the other. Remembering the lessons of history is crucial to make sure that Rwanda, Kosovo, the Holocaust, the killing fields of Cambodia are never repeated. It is in our hands to teach ourselves and our children. We choose what we teach the next generation. The alternative is the Protestant toddler in Northern Ireland with a T-shirt printed with the logo *Born to walk down the Garvahey Road*. Before he can even speak, he is being taught that his inheritance is one of hatred and confrontation. That kind of hatred should make us catch our breath and wonder at the world we would have our children inherit.

The solution for what is happening in the world lies with us as individuals. If we can learn the lessons of our own history, if we can really come to forgiveness for the events and traumas in our own lives and truly let go of them, we will become islands of peace in the world. Eventually that will have a ripple effect throughout the world. But remembering the lessons of our own personal history is central to the journey of forgiveness. If you don't learn from what has happened to you, then you are in danger of it happening again.

If we open the window of forgiveness, even a crack, to acknowledge that it is a good idea, it then follows that all must be forgivable. Not that we must or should forgive—that is a path for each of us to walk—but that it is possible. Sometimes it takes us a long time to be ready to learn the lessons of history in our own individual lives. Until we do, we are stuck, unable to change, rerunning the same film over and over again in our heads. Yet the lack of forgiveness continues to connect us to the act and to the perpetrator. The invisible elastic of hatred binds us closer and closer together. There is something in the ability to forgive and remember even the most despicable acts that cuts the connection.

Tomas Borge, a Nicaraguan Sandinista fighter, captured by the Contras and brutally tortured, understood that. Confronting his torturer after the war had ended, the court entitled him to name the punishment appropriate for his torturer. Borge responded, "My punishment is to forgive you."

It is not "forgive and forget" as if nothing wrong had ever happened, but "forgive and go forward," building on the mistakes of the past and the energy generated by reconciliation to create a new future.

CAROLYN OSIEK

A tribal exercise in challenging your preconceptions

We spend much of our lives categorizing and judging people we don't know because it makes us comfortable to recognize our own tribes and to literally put others in their place. If it comes to a fight, we feel that we will immediately know where we stand.

Spend today noticing all the tribes you encounter and how they make you feel. Try this exercise out on public transportation, at a restaurant, or a gas station.

What group does the person next to you belong to? How can you tell? And how do you judge the person accordingly?

Some examples:

Private school
Projects
Single mother
Alcoholic
Brat

What newspaper is the person reading and how does that affect your judgment of the person? What clothes is the person wearing— and does that make a difference?

Notes

[1] *Sunday Times*, 8 August 1999

[2] Rowe, Dorothy, *Friends and Enemies: Our Need to Love and Hate* (Harper Collins, 2000)

[3] Ignatieff, Michael, *The Warrior's Honor* (Chatto and Windus), p. 330

[4] For more information about the Corrymeela community visit the Web site—www.corrymeela.org

[5] Wiesenthal, Simon, *The Sunflower: On the Possibilities and Limits of Forgiveness*, edited by Harry James Cargas and Bonny V. Fetterman (Schocken Books, 1998), p. 25

[6] Ibid, p. 53

[7] Ibid, p. 53

[8] Ibid, p. 65

[9] Ibid, p. 119

[10] www.journeyofhope.org

[11] Murder Victims' Families for Reconciliation (www.mvfr.org)—an invaluable Web site with many good links

9

Everyday Forgiveness:
The Ongoing Journey

Nothing worth doing is completed in our lifetime; therefore
we are saved by hope.

Nothing true or beautiful or good makes complete sense in any
immediate context of history; therefore we are saved by faith.

Nothing we do, however virtuous, can be accomplished
alone; therefore we are saved by love.

No virtuous act is quite as virtuous from the standpoint of our
friend or foe as from our own; therefore we are saved by the
final form of love, which is forgiveness.

REINHOLD NIEBUHR

"*When you know better, you do better.*" With these words, Maya
Angelou has defined the essence of taking forgiveness
into the ongoing journey of our lives. So now that you do know
better, what difference is it going to make in your daily life? Time
to take the lessons of the Forgiveness Formula into your present
and future.

We have examined the reasons we need to forgive and what happens when we don't. We have practiced forgiveness with the easy

list of people who have hurt us. We have begun to make inroads into the hard list of people who have done us serious wrong.

We have acknowledged how withholding forgiveness keeps us stuck in the past. When we are stuck there, it is like rerunning a film of our lives that is on a loop, so we never get to see the next reel.

Forgiveness allows us to change the reel and enjoy the rest of the film. Using the Forgiveness Room and different visualizations, we have the tools to look at our forgiveness issues and let them go. Now we have to take what we have learned into our present and future.

The Forgiveness Room was a place of safety, somewhere to learn how to let go. It can get to feel so comfortable that it feels like a place of refuge we don't want to leave. But the Forgiveness Room needs to become simply another place in your heart, like love or gratitude—there when you need it, but not a place where you need to hide from the outside world. It is time to step out of the room and into the active rough and tumble of your life.

Just because you know how forgiveness works doesn't mean that the issue will go away. But there's no need to worry. One thing you can be sure of is that life will continue to throw situations at you just so you can check out how you are doing in the forgiveness stakes!

Peggy thought she had "figured out forgiveness. I understood what my core issues of forgiveness were and I had worked through the people on my lists. Then I went into work one day and found I had a new boss—who was a living nightmare. She pressed just about every forgiveness button I had. Suddenly I felt I was right back where I started."

In fact Peggy had learned enough to recognize what was happening—a vital first step in ongoing forgiveness. This new boss wanted someone to fight with, to establish her authority over the office. The "aha" moment of awareness means you don't immediately go in all guns blazing. You have enough distance to evaluate the situation.

"Although I found her hard work—she was always on my case, asking the impossible, while doing very little herself—I knew this was about me, not her. I could choose if I wanted to fight or not. I chose to forgive her.

So I'd go into work every day thinking, I forgive you for all you are going to try to do to hurt me today. As soon as I did, she lost the ability to plunge me straight back into wanting to fight. I was powerful again. I'd go to the bathroom, get a coffee, go out for a quick walk around the block, anything to break the atmosphere she created. Amazingly it worked! She soon moved on to targeting someone else—someone who was prepared to fight."

This is what moving out of the safety of the Forgiveness Room into the whirlwind of your life means. You can trust your forgiveness judgment. Armed with the Forgiveness Formula you are safe. Let's just look at the formula again:

- It means completely letting go of the hurt this person has done you.
- It means letting go of the hold this narrative has had on your life.
- It means getting rid of a piece of baggage that you will no longer have to carry around with you.
- It does not mean forgetting what has been done to you.
- It does not mean that you do not learn lessons from what happened to you.

Just because you have been through your forgiveness lists and understood what your deep underlying issues with forgiveness have been, doesn't mean that you won't have to practice forgiveness in the future. In fact, to begin with it may seem that people are trying to test out the new you, in the same way that when you give up smoking or drinking, some people are always trying to get you to fall off the wagon.

But you've got your forgiveness license now—you've passed the test. Remember the first time you drove on the highway, how fast all the cars seemed to be going? Ongoing forgiveness is just like that. Keep practicing on a daily basis, resolving issues as you go along and soon you'll be happy to pull into the fast lane.

Ongoing forgiveness means a daily workout. People will come and test you, bump up against your issues. Now you know what they are, you know they are *your issues* and you can see the tests as just that—seeing how well you are doing with forgiveness. Let them go and you will be astonished at how much better you feel in your everyday life. No more stored resentments, no buildups of anger, no more churning stomachs with tension and stress.

That's not to say that sometimes it won't be hard. When you have looked at your core issues of forgiveness and dealt with them, they will begin to lose their power. But until you resolve them completely, you will still feel a twinge, like any old injury, when someone comes along and presses that button for you. The key to not reverting back to our harmful default settings with forgiveness is space. Forgiveness gives you the space to see them coming and not react as you would have done in the past. The space to allow enough distance between someone pressing our core issue buttons and diving straight back into the old ways of reacting.

Chloe, who used to let her family pattern of bearing grudges dominate her relationships, now feels completely different. "*Now I don't behave in the same way. Learning to forgive has really made a difference. I don't* start building up a grudge. I look at the situation, like in the Forgiveness Room when you tell the person, then you let the person speak, and then you stand back and then they speak together. . . . that is what I would do now."

Making it happen . . . resolve to do things differently

You can't change the way people behave, but you can change the way you react. Resolve to be different, to figure out anything that comes up as you go along. Not to let it fester until it becomes more important and significant than it needs to be. Remember that you are allowed to get it wrong sometimes. No one's perfect. But just as you need to forgive, you have to be prepared to ask for forgiveness too.

A close friend called while I was writing this chapter and without thinking I picked up the phone. I was distracted and wanted to get back to work, but rather than say that, I half listened to what she was saying, hoping the conversation would end soon. She was telling me about what had been going on in her life since the last time we spoke; I was thinking how much I wanted to get on with writing. When we eventually put the phone down, I turned back to my work with relief, feeling slightly uncomfortable that I hadn't really wanted to talk at all but hadn't admitted it. I knew that I hadn't been present in that phone call and I felt bad. So an hour later I called and explained and apologized. She laughed and forgave me. It was worked out—gone.

Learning to deal with forgiveness in your everyday life is just like any new skill. If you have decided to get fit, you know that you have to commit to your decision on a daily basis—it's that extra walk or run or flight of stairs that is money in your fitness bank account. Forgiveness is just the same: practice it every day and it will become as familiar as brushing your teeth. Some people find that the end of the day is a good time to do a quick run-through of events. Is there anyone you need to forgive for what they did to you today? Or do you need forgiveness? Think how you can put it right tomorrow.

> One must put oneself in everyone's position. To understand everything is to forgive everything.
>
> TOLSTOY

If someone has hurt you badly during the day, it may be helpful to make a quick list, to show you what your real feelings are about the situation:

I could forgive if . . .

If I don't forgive . . .

The chance to practice is all around you

Just as you notice a new word everywhere you look when you have learned its meaning, so it is with forgiveness—you will see it in a new light in many of your relationships, either with people who are very good or terrible at it, or others who can't bear the subject to come up. Chloe has found that her way of being in the world has changed radically since she started being serious about dealing with forgiveness. It's as though she has put on a new pair of glasses—she literally sees her relationships in a different focus. "OK, *I've gotten annoyed, I've been upset by somebody, but then my mind will start think-ing, 'What about the other person's point of view?' Then I will start thinking, 'Forget my point of view, forget the other person's point of view, what is the effect that keeping that grudge would have into the future? Do I want to take it there?' And the answer is always no! It's really worked for me, it's been a big change."*

Work in progress . . .

Now you have grasped what forgiveness really entails there are certain pointers you may find helpful:

- Don't beat yourself up if you get it wrong sometimes.
- Treat each day as a clean slate.
- The more practice you get, the more fluent you'll get.
- Trust the process.

The further you travel along the forgiveness road, the more you will recognize that we are all "works in progress." If you trust the process, you will find yourself behaving differently, which will mean that everything else around you will change, too. Pretty soon you will be surprised at how differently you can react and how that has a domino effect in your relationships in everyday life.

Recently I was at a meeting and bumped into a friend I hadn't seen in ages. We chatted and came to some stairs. As I have a bad ankle, I need to look down and be careful on stairs. My friend was right behind me. As I got to the bottom of the stairs, someone caught my eye and needed to talk to me urgently. When I turned around, the friend I hadn't seen for ages had disappeared. Funny, I thought, maybe he didn't want to talk after all. Oh, well, too bad. By the time I got home, I had a nice little grudge beginning to simmer on the back boiler. Here was someone I hadn't seen in ages, I thought of him as a friend and had wanted to catch up with him and he had disappeared. Some friend! But a doubt lingered in my mind . . . so I e-mailed him and got an e-mail right back.

It turned out he had gone off because he felt guilty about not getting in touch and thought I was ignoring him (not knowing about my bad ankle nor having noticed the other person claim my attention).

This is a classic everyday misunderstanding, where both people feel hurt and are not sure what to do next—fertile ground for grudge growing. The one thing you shouldn't do is leave it and hope things will work themselves out. I shot an e-mail straight back and explained about the bad ankle, the other person having caught my eye, and my surprise at his disappearance. How you word your attempt at reconciliation is crucial—tone is everything. I could have blamed him for not waiting but I realized this was just a misunderstanding and that we were both slightly hurt.

Did I need to be right or did I want to see this person I really liked and reconnect? If you can stop in your tracks and ask that question in your daily life, you will be able to nip most conflicts in the bud. Next day I met my friend in the street and we laughed about the misunderstanding and arranged to meet again. Our friendship was all the stronger for it. Silence and hurt feelings are ideal growing conditions for new grudges. Feed them with unspoken resentment, water with loving care, and pretty soon you can have a fully grown grudge flowering in your heart.

Getting to the heart of the matter . . .

Acknowledging your part in conflicts that will arise in your everyday life leaves you open to the possibility of being hurt, which is something we all try to avoid wherever possible. In fact, owning up to having messed up allows the other person to come toward you; after all, would you stay on your high horse if someone took the blame for what was really just crossed wires? It is not a question of trying to apportion blame, but of getting to the real truth of a situation.

In any misunderstanding you might like to ask yourself some questions:

- ❧ What did I do to contribute to this?
- ❧ How can I let go?
- ❧ What would a third party say if he or she could see the situation and knew all the facts?

We need to be able to tolerate ambiguity. Maybe a situation has more than one interpretation—ours? It's useful to put yourself in the other person's shoes for a moment: how would they tell the story? If all else fails and you are still struggling with whose fault it is, with getting your version of the truth acknowledged, try the acid test of forgiveness:

"If I knew I had twenty-four hours left to live, would this matter?"

Pierre is a respected member of a small village community in France and he understands that the sooner a potential conflict is nipped in the bud, the better.

"*The mayor of our tiny village in France changed after many years. It had always been in the hands of the powerful landowners, but now it had changed so that a small farmer became mayor. There was a lot of strong feeling in the village and the first meeting of the new village council was a stormy one. The old mayor grudgingly handed over* power to the new one and as is the tradition, after the meeting everyone went to the bar for a drink. There the argument flared up again and the old mayor suddenly slapped the new one in full view of everyone else."

Pierre wasn't there to witness the argument, but when he heard about it, he knew it was very serious. In a village of this size, that sort of argument can last for generations, with children and grand-children no longer speaking to one another for some half-remembered bit of land, or argument when those who had it are long dead. Pierre had seen too many similar incidents in the past and knew he had to act quickly.

"So I went to see the old mayor, who had slapped the new one. He was already feel-ing awkward about what had happened and regretted what he had done in the heat of the moment. I told him that if he didn't act right away to put things right, this was a feud that could go on for generations and that it wouldn't be good for the village.

He agreed with me and said something that surprised me. 'I shall have to go and settle this and ask him to forgive me.' He asked me to be the go-between as he wasn't sure what reaction he would get. I contacted the man who had been slapped and they agreed to meet at his house the following Saturday. I wasn't there, but they both told me about it. The man who had done the slapping apologized and asked for forgiveness, they shook hands and it was finished. Then they went back to the same bar and bought each other a drink to publicly show the argument was over. And that was the end of it."

What's interesting about Pierre's account is that the forgiveness took place almost immediately, before bitterness and rancor had had time to set in. Both men trusted Pierre enough to resolve the problem and the former mayor was willing to admit that he had made a mistake and to risk being hurt by asking for forgiveness.

What Pierre shows too is that forgiveness is not about judging. He simply encouraged both sides to come together and let them deal with it.

Not allowing new grudges to take hold is the key. Keep the channels of communication open. It really is as simple as that. We tend to put ourselves at the center of everything without realizing that we all have our own scripts of pain and expectations of how others may hurt us.

When a flare-up happens or feels like it might happen, ask yourself these simple questions:

- What is this really about?
- Does it matter?
- Can I do things differently?

You will find yourself reading from your familiar script of how things have happened in the past. Or the way things "always go." But so is the other person. Neither of you is in the present. You are both acting out past situations of hurt.

Making forgiveness happen means putting that old script down and choosing to act differently now. Remember:

- I can choose to act differently.
- I can't change the other person, but I can change the way I react.
- When I change, everything is different.

You'll be astonished that when you change, the other person will change too in ways that will surprise you. Forgiveness is like a dance: if you start dancing a waltz instead of a foxtrot, the other person is going to look pretty silly if he or she insists on staying with the foxtrot even though the music has changed.

You have a choice in each new situation that life throws at you. Treat each day as a new start in your life of forgiveness—you've got the new tracksuit and trainers, now get out there and run!

For Chloe, making it happen is about not taking the learned script into her everyday relationships as she used to. *"It's back to the dialogue in the Forgiveness Room, really learning to express why someone has hurt you and when you really look at it, then you realize that it's totally dependent on you, therefore you can do something to change it. I'm really able to let go; it's difficult though and it's continuous and you can't do it once and for all. I am very quick-tempered and I will get irritated if I don't get what I want or if things don't happen my way but I'm much faster at realizing it. I'm better at forgiving myself now too. I've started, but it will take time."*

Sometimes the immediate family narrative is too familiar to change easily. We can, without realizing it, take the prime issues of the difficult relationships of the hard list into all our other relationships, even when it's not applicable or appropriate.

Chris has realized that it is all too easy to take the learned family script—withdrawal and silence—into other relationships with friends and partners, when that is inappropriate. *"I tend to withdraw from situations with sulky silence. It doesn't work at all, it's a really crappy way of dealing with it. It shows people that I'm pissed off, but generally people don't know why I'm pissed off. It took me a very long time to realize that they just see it as sulky and really don't connect it at all. So I do try these days to make it clearer what is connected with what."*

Of course the hard list throws up issues that will continually appear in our journey of forgiveness. Many of the people involved will still be in our lives: partners, parents, siblings. This list combines our core issues with some of the most testing people in our lives; because they are our most intimate relationships, this is where our struggles are most intensely felt and magnified. How do we deal with them in the ongoing journey?

Chloe recognized this recently and was pleased that she didn't react in the way she once would have done. *"The one I'm working on at the moment is my dad. The funny thing is that there is a new grudge that could have built up with my dad's sister following my grandmother's funeral. But I have just let it go. I'm actually able to stop any grudges building up because of what I have learned. It's given me the tools to cope."*

Struggle or dance?

We have a choice in each new relationship to take the familiar hurt into the future or let it go. Chris is working on being different with her husband. She is developing a new narrative with him that she also wants to pass on to her child. Being conscious of your inherited pattern is more than half the battle—you can simply decide to be different. *"We have to not interact very much for a few hours and then it's fine. In the past the argument would have ended but not been resolved and it would have come up again the next time we argued. It is great that we don't bring up past arguments and that's a very big departure for me."*

That doesn't mean it won't be a struggle to escape the narrative that is firmly embedded in your consciousness. Or that your family won't try to bring you back into the fold: after all, if you call a halt to the script, stop struggling, and start dancing, it means they no longer get to play the same games—but just saying it out loud admits the possibility of change. As Chris has found with her husband: *"We often talk and talk about something and then it just dies ... and we have really let go of it. But this is the first relationship, I'd say, where that is the case. We talk and talk and talk, and it's let go because it feels like there is nowhere to go with it. I would definitely have borne a grudge in other relationships. But in this one, the way we talk about it does seem to work in that we do seem to be able to talk about it and really let it go."*

If an issue has really been dealt with, it doesn't need to be resurrected every time there is conflict. We will always have our arguments with our nearest and dearest, but the danger in these fights is the unspoken subtext of unhappiness—get it out in the open and it can be examined, discussed, and resolved.

The good news about forgiveness in our lives is that it has a ripple effect. If you get forgiveness right in one relationship, you will quickly see the benefits and understand how much easier life could be if you applied the same approach to other, more problematic relationships.

Betty has abandoned the imaginary little black book where she used to store all the bad things her boyfriends did. Rather than discussing the issue, a day would come when the tally would be overwhelming and they would find themselves ex-boyfriends without really understanding why. *"I don't do that anymore because I realized that a good relationship means that you discuss these issues. If a relationship is worth staying in, whether it is a friend or partner, you discuss them and you hear what the other person has got to say. I think forgiving is a really good thing to do; it's like letting go of a great weight. While you are at a point where it is difficult, it usually means you keep going back to the period or the incident that made you resentful in the first place. If I can decide that it's over then I can let it go."*

> Life is an adventure in forgiveness.
> NORMAN COUSINS

It may be that you are the first in your family prepared to do things differently. Being different can feel dangerous and isolating, but it gives everyone else a chance to be different too. If you refuse to play the family narrative, then the ripple effect will surprise you.

Why some people seem to be chosen to change the family pattern is a mystery. Through a different education or chance sequence of events in their lives, they suddenly see the family pattern of forgiveness for what it is and then seek to change it. This was what Tina found in her life. She became the person who asked questions in her family and although that was initially very difficult for everyone, it has meant that she has not perpetuated the family narrative of grudges.

"I wanted to change it; from as early as I could remember I wanted to change things. And make them better. I fundamentally love them and care about them. I began to understand that there was no point in holding onto grudges. Because even though I hadn't processed it all, I had an instinctive understanding of these sorts of dynamics even as a very young child. I knew intuitively that it didn't work to hold those grudges. It hadn't ever worked in what I knew of my family on both sides."

Our forgiveness issues can also leak into our professional lives. Tony had a major core issue with his brother as a child and found himself reproducing that relationship at work. *"In the past I looked for the same situation and played out the same old drama over and over again. In my first job I found myself a manager who had a similar character to my brother and it led to the situation where I started fighting against him, not realizing he was my superior. I can tell you it brought me an awful lot of trouble. I did the same thing with my second employer, but that time I connected to a man who looked like my father. Even my ex-wife had a character I now can tell is a lot like my brother."*

So how have things changed for Tony, now he has forgiven and let go of his brother and his parents? *"Today I think, after all the pain I have been through, I can let go of these kinds of issues, take an attitude of not responding or reacting in many situations. This is not completely to my satisfaction because I still withdraw or don't respond on many occasions."*

When we change we can expect to scare some of the people around us. Most people like to think they know you once and for all and what your reactions will be in certain situations. So when your narrative of forgiveness changes, some of those people will not be able to go forward with you into your new life. There is no blame attached—you just grow out of some people. They were right for one phase of your life; now they aren't right for you and you aren't right for them.

Letting go of those people in your life who no longer fit

A certain amount of clearing out of your address book may become necessary—some of those people who have been in your life will no longer seem appropriate.

Linda, who was bullied as a child by her two brothers and used anger as her main defense, feels forgiveness has brought her enough distance to call a halt to the immediate cause and effect. She no longer uses other people as a punching bag for her past. "I don't react so strongly now and if I do lose my temper, I'm less likely to try and justify it to myself. Before, I would go straight for the 'no jury in the land would convict you' approach!"

She has found that some of her friends have not been able to cope with her new persona and is surprised to discover that they liked the angry Linda but can't cope with the new calmer version. Linda has found it hard to let go of some of those people, who have turned out not to be the good friends she thought they were, because they are unwilling to recognize that she has changed.

Sometimes our change of heart makes people uncomfortable. It is as though we are somehow holding up a mirror to their own lives and issues of forgiveness. And if we can change so dramatically, where does that leave them?

We saw in an earlier chapter that we teach people how to treat us. While their treatment of us may have been acceptable in the past, once we have found our way on the path of forgiveness, that may have consequences for many of our relationships. You may have to say goodbye, while wishing them well, in order to be able to go forward in your new view of life.

There is a great Nina Simone song, "Don't Smoke in Bed," in which she sings about writing a man a letter to tell him she is leaving; she ends each verse with "don't smoke in bed." You can still care for someone even as you are walking out of the door.

Don't worry if you get it wrong sometimes. The past you is a pattern of thoughts and ideas that you have carefully constructed and is familiar. The danger is that in any crisis you may default back to the same way of dealing with pain. Even though it doesn't work and you know that, it is your default pattern and that is the most difficult pattern to break. You have to do it consciously. Take yourself back into the Forgiveness Room regularly and do a forgiveness inventory on your hard list—and don't forget yourself.

Laura has made a new life for herself with her two children; she's divorced from the husband who used to bully her. They are still in contact because of the children, but forgiveness has brought her a new way of dealing with him that works much better.

"Quite often if he does something that annoys me, it's because I am grasping back at my old sense of identity, someone who was hurt or damaged by him or undermined by him. But if I actually get off that kind of circular thinking and say to myself— is this really a problem from my current perspective of someone who is happy with her life?—then I am in a position to say that either it is not a problem at all, or if it is a problem, then I deal with it and say, 'No, this isn't ok,' or whatever. So it's ongoing, but it is a continual decision whether or not to get on that circular thinking, reconstructing this harmed, damaged, and undermined self any more or just to say, 'No, that's not me, I don't need to do that.'"

Eventually you will recognize the pattern and loop and be able to say, "Oh here we are again," like greeting someone you used to know and you haven't seen for a long time.

If it is a core issue it will come back and visit, in different forms and in different people until you deal with it and it loses its power. And even then it remains a scar. The issue will come up under the guise of different people, just to see if you want to go back to the old ways, which, however uncomfortable they are, remain familiar and are as tempting as a favorite old sweater.

The fact that we have a choice when it comes to forgiveness is a powerful force for good in our lives. When we recognize this, we lose our victim status. Although it is not a simple decision and the choice to engage with the process of forgiveness will undoubtedly change our lives beyond recognition, it will, in the end, be a change for the better. Tina has understood this at a profound level. *"Forgiveness is a very tender thing and it only really works when you can let go of any hurt that you feel. It's a choice that I can make in my life to let go of the hurts and forgive so that I can be free. The strongest piece of advice that I would give to anybody is to be free to live their life as consciously and as well as they can. To be free, you have to be able to forgive."*

Chloe recognizes that forgiveness has softened her heart both toward the outside world and herself. In the past she was most hard on herself; now she is learning to be more gentle—and it shows. *"My spirit is lighter because of it; I can really concentrate on what is important today and what I want to achieve. There is no comparison, I'm just happier."*

We are responsible for the forgiveness narrative in our lives. We can change the narrative that we have been handed down the generations. One of the things we have seen is that we can only expect to change ourselves in this journey of forgiveness. But if we do change, everything around us will change, too. So do you want to be an instrument of peace or of conflict? It is up to you.

> Do you want to be happy for a moment? Then seek revenge.
> Do you want to be happy for ever? Then grant forgiveness.
>
> HENRI LACORDAIRE

Individual gestures of forgiveness can have great significance for the world. Nelson Mandela inviting his jailer to his inauguration as president of South Africa sent a ripple of astonishment across the world. And those gestures may take many different forms. In September 1999 the first concert on German soil by the Israeli Philharmonic Orchestra playing with a German orchestra took place. Beneath the hill at Buchenwald, Zubin Mehta conducted more than 170 musicians only hours after many of them had visited the Nazi extermination camp where more than 50,000 people died.

"The thought did run through my mind at the camp: how will Israelis be able to sit together with Germans this evening and play music?" Mehta said. *"But I detected no feelings of resistance."*

Let us not underestimate the difficulty. I know from my own experience of abduction that forgiveness can take years to address. I buried the memory, then told someone and felt it had been put to rest. But it resurfaced strongly again and I realized that the hatred and bitterness were still there, buried deep within my heart—that feeling so much hatred for this man, being willing to kill him, would eventually poison all my other relationships.

It has taken a long time, but I know now that I have let him go completely. Forgiven him. The domino effect in my life is spectacular

—forgiveness has freed me to be different in all my other relationships.

It is a path that can bring so much pain to the surface that we may have to pause several times along the journey. It can seem sometimes that too much is being asked of us. There is no rush. We have taken a lifetime to get to where we are; there is plenty of time for us to come to forgiveness. But each decision we make to walk along the difficult path of forgiveness is like a light shining in the darkness.

Luke, who was sexually abused, has been transformed by forgiving himself and his abuser. He has changed so much and the domino effects in his life have been so radical that he has become a different person altogether.

"I can put my hand on my heart and say that I am more of a free man today than I have ever been. Does that mean that I have almost completed the journey? I don't know: all I know is that I have begun the journey and that is what is important."

We have choices in our ongoing life of forgiveness. Life will continue to throw difficult situations and people at us. We may have to face terrible times that seem beyond our power to forgive. But we always have a choice: do I choose to struggle or dance?

Nelson Mandela shows us the difference forgiveness can make in a life. Not just at a personal level, but out in the world. We have seen only too starkly the ripple effects of revenge and hatred in the world. We know where that leads. So do we dare to do things differently? While we may be scared to forgive and let go of the past, if we can summon the courage to make that journey, the repercussions for peace in the world are immense. If you take a step toward forgiveness, the world is transformed.

Last year I went out for a meal with some friends. It wasn't until halfway through dinner that I realized that for the first time in my life, I was sitting with my back to the door. Forgiving my abductor had finally made me feel safe.

Our deepest fear is not that we are inadequate. Our deepest fear is that we are powerful beyond measure. It is our Light, not our Darkness, that most frightens us.

We ask ourselves, "Who am I to be brilliant, gorgeous, talented and fabulous?" Actually, who are you not to be? You are a child of God; your playing small doesn't serve the world . . . We were born to make manifest the glory of God within us. It is not just in some of us, it is in everyone and as we let our own light shine we unconsciously give other people permission to do the same. As we are liberated from our own fear, our presence automatically liberates others.

MARIANNE WILLIAMSON

Forgiveness is the key to all our futures. It opens a whole new world of possibilities for us all.

To forgive is to say, "It stops here. Now. With me."

Forgiveness Workshops

*I*F YOU WOULD like more information about forgiveness workshops that are based on the material in this book, please e-mail timetoforgive@hotmail.com.

Bibliography

Estes, Clarissa Pinkola, *Women Who Run with the Wolves* (Rider, 1992)

Foundation for Inner Peace, *A Course in Miracles* (Arkana, 1997)

Henderson, Michael, *Forgiveness: Breaking the Chain of Hate* (Grosvenor Books, 2002)

Ignatieff, Michael, *The Warrior's Honor* (Chatto and Windus)

Kornfeld, Jack, *A Path with Heart: A Guide Through the Perils and Promises of Spiritual Life* (Rider, 1994)

Kübler-Ross, Elizabeth, and Kessler, David, *Life Lessons: Two Experts on Death and Dying Teach Us About the Mysteries of Life and Living* (Simon and Schuster, 2000)

Monbourquette, John, *How to Forgive: A Step-by-Step Guide* (Darton Longman and Todd, 2000)

Rowe, Dorothy, *Friends and Enemies: Our Need to Love and Hate* (Harper-Collins, 2000)

Tutu, Desmond, *No Future Without Forgiveness* (Rider, 1999)

Wiesenthal, Simon, *The Sunflower: On the Possibilities and Limits of Forgiveness*, edited by Harry James Cargas and Bonny V. Fetterman (Schocken Books, 1998)

Acknowledgments

THIS BOOK WOULD never have seen the light of day without the support and encouragement of my family and friends. A big thank you to Monique Griffin, Tim and Isobel Griffin, Francoise Griffin, and Christopher Beale. A special thank you to Emma, Tommy, Luke, Ellen, Ellie, and Rebecca, who reminded me that there was still a lot of fun to be had out there in the world.

Special thanks to my friends who talked through the issues with me and just listened when I needed to talk—thanks to Mary Rose Tarpey, Mary Ambrose, Camilla de Crespigny, Tim Salmon, Kath Hopkins, Father Robert Plourde, Peter and Marian Daglish, Doris Stubbs, Father Pat Browne, James Parker, Fiona Hill, Hazel Castell, Jill Burridge, Tony James, Sarah Bushman. I couldn't have done it without you.

A big bouquet of thank-yous to Miranda Birch, who read through many of the chapters and brought her invaluable criticism and encouragement in the last difficult months.

Thanks to the Findhorn Foundation, whose Forgiveness conference was a revelation. Thanks also to Anne Slack, who helped me start on the road of my own forgiveness; to Dr. Elizabeth Muir, who saw me through some rough water; and to Philip Allen, osteopath, who was there through the whole process.

I'd also like to thank my agent, Jane Judd, and the editor of the U.K. edition at Simon and Schuster, Helen Gummer, who believed in the book from the beginning. Thanks also to Cassandra Campbell and Catherine Hurley for their sterling work on the editing of the U.K. edition of the book.

Finally I'd like to thank all those people who were willing to share their experiences of forgiveness with me with such generosity and openness.